Easy Vegan Cookbook

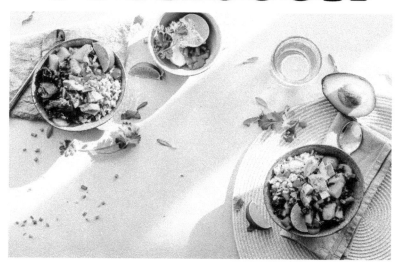

Discover The Benefits of Eating a Plant Based Diet with Quick and Delicious Illustrated Recipes for Weight Loss and Healthier Living. Change Your Nutrition Plan and Feel Great!

Jeremy Tayler

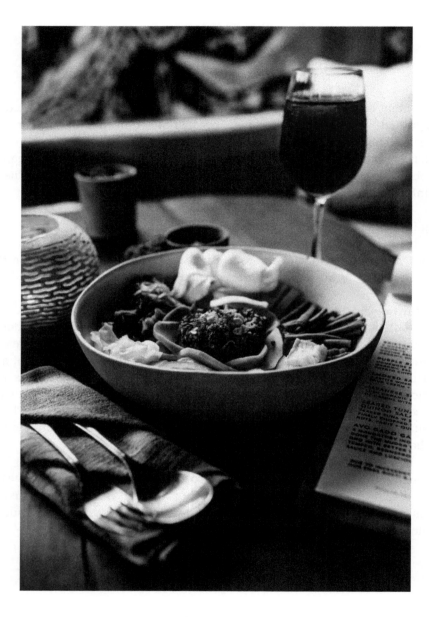

Let's Start!

Table of Contents

BLT Summer Rolls with Avocado
Perfect Roasted Potatoes
Cauliflower Alfredo Baked Ziti
Creamy Roasted Garlic–Tomato Soup with Grilled Cheese Croutons
Chocolate–Peanut Butter Truffles

GAME DAY VEGAN
Buffalo Cauliflower Wings with Blue Cheese Dip
Jalapeño Popper Bites
Cheesy Spiced Popcorn
Chickpea-Avocado Taquitos
Pizzadillas
Cilantro Chile Almond Dip

GET-TOGETHER VEGAN MEALS
Avocado & Hearts of Palm Tea Sandwiches
Roasted Red Pepper Hummus Cucumber Cups
Chickpea Caesar Pasta Salad
Sun-Dried Tomato & White Bean Bruschetta
Chickpea Croquettes with Dill Yogurt Sauce
Champagne Cupcakes

VEGAN BARBEQUES
Deviled Potato Salad
Herbed Tofu Burgers
Ranch-Seasoned Corn on the Cob
Creamy, Crunchy Coleslaw
Grilled Veggie Kebabs
Rainbow Fruit Salad with Maple-Lime Dressing

VEGAN HOLIDAYS
Cheesy Roasted Sweet Potatoes
Green Bean Casserole with Crispy Onion Topping
Mashed Potatoes
Maple-Miso Tempeh Cutlets
Easy Tahini Gravy
Marbled Pumpkin Cheesecake
Gingerbread Cookies

VEGANIZED FAMILY FAVORITES
Tempeh Sausage Minestrone
Pot-obello Roast
Sweet Potato Casserole
Skillet Cornbread
Grandma's Famous Date Nut Bread
Peanut Butter Pie

ROMANTIC VEGAN
Silky Cheese Fondue
Avocado, Pomegranate & Pine Nut Salad
Deconstructed Sushi Bowl
Sun-Dried Tomato Linguine
Scallops with Creamy Mushroom-Leek Sauce
Mini Salted Chocolate Caramel Pretzel Tarts

VEGAN HOMEMADE EDIBLE GIFTS
Rescue Puppy Chow
Caramel Cashew Granola
Wild Rice, Mushroom & Lentil Soup in a Jar
Make-Your-Own Cornbread in a Jar
Apricot Pistachio Chocolate Bark
Spiced Nuts

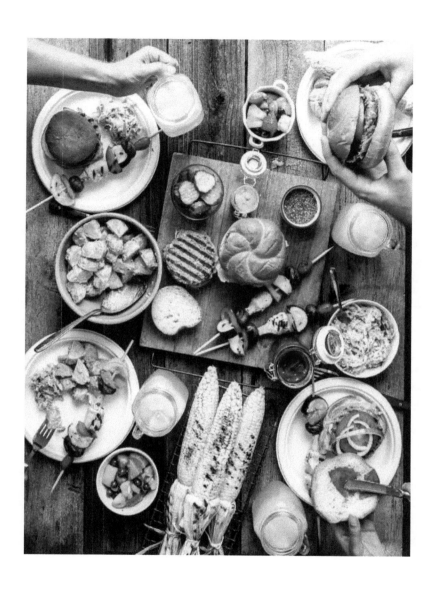

VEGAN STAPLES

Quick Bacon Crumbles
Basic Cashew Cheese Sauce
Pepita Parmesan
Pickled Red Cabbage & Onion Relish
Cream of Mushroom Soup
Avocado Ranch Dressing
Lemon Tahini Sauce

VEGAN BREAKFAST

Tofu Rancheros
Maple–Peanut Butter Pancakes
Savory Breakfast Casserole
Everyone's Favorite Oatmeal
Vanilla French Toast with Strawberry Sauce
Mushroom-Kale Skillet Hash
Quick & Easy Avocado Toast

EASY VEGAN WEEKSNIGHTS

Tips & Tricks: Weeknight Meal Preparation
Mexican Pizza with 15-Minute Refried Beans
Potato Leek Soup
Quick Cauliflower Curry
BBQ Chickpea Salad
Spicy Sesame Soba Noodle Bowl
Cheesy Quinoa & Veggies
Jackfruit Crabless Cakes with Lemon Dill Aïoli

KID FRIENDLY VEGAN

Hidden Veggie Mac 'n' Cheese
Tempeh Nuggets
Cheesy Trees
PB&J Roll-Ups
Fruity Granola Bars
Bean & Cheese Quesadillas

VEGAN SNACKS & FINGER FOODS

Make-Your-Own Cheese Pizza
Smashed Lentil Tacos
Tempeh Sloppy Joe Sliders
Tater Totchos
Just Fries
Hot Fudge Ice Cream Sundaes

THE FAVORITES - VEGAN STYLE

Cheese-Stuffed Meatballs
Ultimate Twice-Baked Potatoes
Double-Double Cheeseburgers
Beer-Marinated Portobello Tacos with Avocado-Corn Salsa
Lazy Vegan Chile Relleno Casserole
Jackfruit Carnitas Burrito Bowl

BALANCED VEGAN

Chinese Chickpea Salad
Pecan Pesto Spaghetti Squash with Peas & Kale
Chile-Roasted Tofu Lettuce Cups
Buddha Bowl
Beet Hummus Collard Wraps
Green Quinoa Salad
No-Bake Zucchini Manicotti

HOMESTYLE VEGAN

Chickpea & Dumplin' Soup
Shiitake Stroganoff
Unstuffed Cabbage Rolls
Not-Tuna Casserole
BBQ-Glazed Tempeh
Smoky Shroom Sausage & Red Potato Goulash

VEGAN CLASSICS

Balsamic-Roasted Beet & Cheese Galette
French Onion Soup
Truffled Mashed Potato–Stuffed Portobellos
Butternut Squash Risotto with Sage Butter
Kung Pao Cauliflower
Creamy Spinach-Artichoke Pasta

VEGAN SANDWICHES

Fillet o' Chickpea Sandwich with Tartar Sauce Slaw
The Portobello Philly Reuben
BBQ Pulled Jackfruit Sandwich
The Avocado Melt
Chickenless Salad Sandwich
Lemongrass Tofu Banh Mi

VEGAN BAKING

Blueberry-Banana Muffins
Chocolate Layer Cake
Peanut Butter Oatmeal Cookies
Salted Vanilla Maple Blondies
Pumpkin Chai Scones
Strawberry-Peach Crisp with Vanilla Whipped Cream

VEGAN COMFORT FOOD

Hash Brown Casserole (aka Company Potatoes)
Roasted Carrot & Wild Mushroom Ragout
Sweet Potato Shepherd's Pie
Lasagna Soup
Cauliflower Parmigiana
Brownie Ice Cream Sandwiches

VEGAN - FOR PICKY EATERS

Artichoke-Kale Hummus
BLT Summer Rolls with Avocado
Perfect Roasted Potatoes
Cauliflower Alfredo Baked Ziti
Creamy Roasted Garlic–Tomato Soup
Chocolate–Peanut Butter Truffles

GAME DAY VEGAN

Buffalo Cauliflower Wings with Blue Cheese Dip
Jalapeño Popper Bites
Cheesy Spiced Popcorn
Chickpea-Avocado Taquitos
Pizzadillas
Cilantro Chile Almond Dip

GET-TOGETHER VEGAN MEALS

Avocado & Hearts of Palm Tea Sandwiches
Roasted Red Pepper Hummus Cucumber Cups
Chickpea Caesar Pasta Salad
Sun-Dried Tomato & White Bean Bruschetta
Chickpea Croquettes with Dill Yogurt Sauce
Champagne Cupcakes

VEGAN BARBEQUES

Deviled Potato Salad
Herbed Tofu Burgers
Ranch-Seasoned Corn on the Cob
Creamy, Crunchy Coleslaw
Grilled Veggie Kebabs
Rainbow Fruit Salad with Maple-Lime Dressing

VEGAN HOLIDAYS

Cheesy Roasted Sweet Potatoes
Green Bean Casserole with Crispy Onion Topping
Mashed Potatoes
Maple-Miso Tempeh Cutlets
Easy Tahini Gravy
Marbled Pumpkin Cheesecake
Gingerbread Cookies

VEGANIZED FAMILY FAVORITES

Tips & Tricks: Veganizing Your Family's Favorite Recipes
Tempeh Sausage Minestrone
Pot-obello Roast
Sweet Potato Casserole
Skillet Cornbread
Grandma's Famous Date Nut Bread
Peanut Butter Pie

ROMANTIC VEGAN

Silky Cheese Fondue
Avocado, Pomegranate & Pine Nut Salad
Deconstructed Sushi Bowl
Sun-Dried Tomato Linguine
Scallops with Creamy Mushroom-Leek Sauce
Mini Salted Chocolate Caramel Pretzel Tarts

VEGAN HOMEMADE EDIBLE GIFTS

Rescue Puppy Chow
Caramel Cashew Granola
Wild Rice, Mushroom & Lentil Soup in a Jar
Make-Your-Own Cornbread in a Jar
Apricot Pistachio Chocolate Bark
Spiced Nuts

9

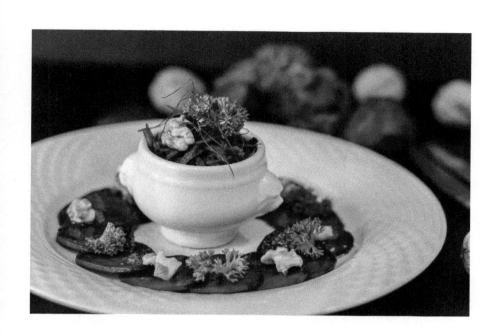

125 Delicious Vegan Illustrated Recipes

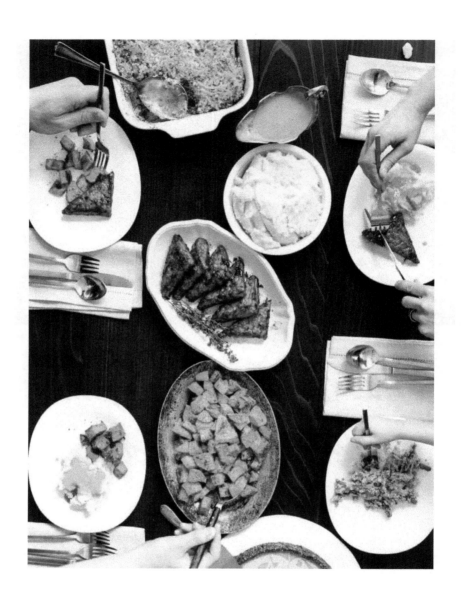

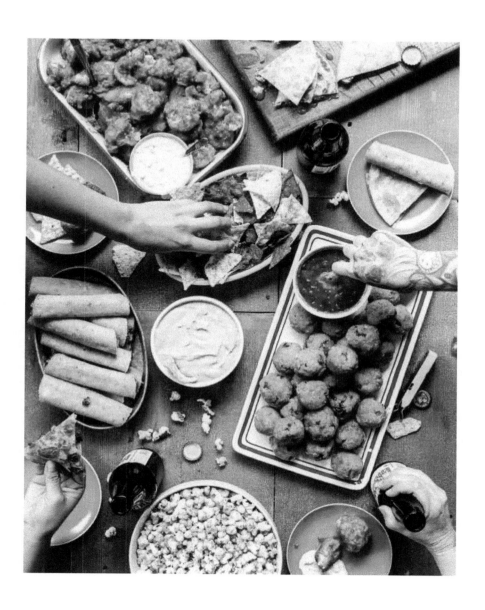

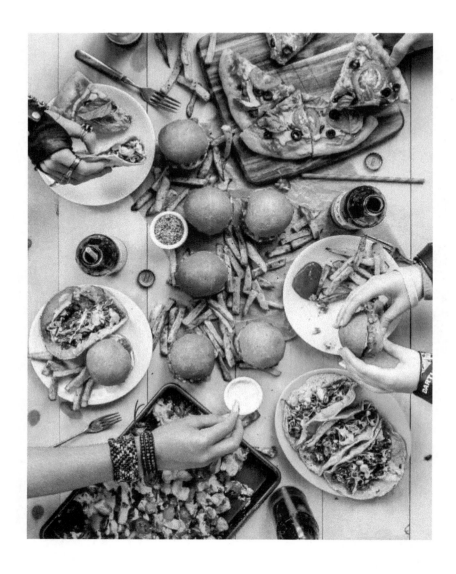

VEGAN STAPLES

VEGAN PANTRY STAPLES THAT YOUR FAMILY WILL BE WILLING TO USE

IN THIS CHAPTER

Quick Bacon Crumbles

MAKES 2 CUPS

PREP TIME: **5 minutes**
ACTIVE TIME: **30 minutes**

One 8-oz. Package tempeh (soy-free if necessary)
¼ cup liquid aminos (or gluten-free tamari; use coconut aminos to be soy-free)
¼ cup low-sodium vegetable broth
2 tablespoons olive oil
1 tablespoon liquid smoke
1 tablespoon maple syrup
½ teaspoon ground cumin
½ teaspoon garlic powder
Black pepper to taste

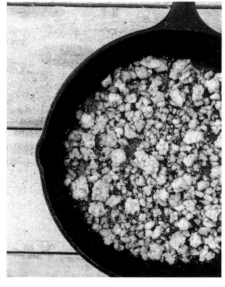

1. Line a plate with paper towels. Crumble the tempeh into small pieces and set aside.

2. Combine the liquid aminos, broth, 1 tablespoon of the olive oil, the liquid smoke, maple syrup, cumin, and garlic powder in a cup. Stir until combined.

3. Heat the remaining olive oil in a large frying pan, preferably cast iron, over medium heat. Add the tempeh crumbles and toss to coat in oil. Cook for about 1 minute, then add the sauce. Cook, stirring every few minutes, until the liquid has been absorbed and the tempeh is tender with a crispy exterior.

4. Transfer the tempeh to the prepared plate to absorb any excess oil. Sprinkle with black pepper. Serve immediately. Leftovers will keep in an airtight container in the fridge for 4 to 5 days.

Basic Cashew Cheese Sauce

MAKES ¾ CUP

PREP	TIME:	5	minutes
ACTIVE	TIME:	10	minutes
INACTIVE TIME:	**60 minutes**		

½ cup raw cashews, soaked in warm water for at least 1 hour and drained, water reserved
5 to 6 tablespoons reserved soaking water
2 tablespoons lemon juice
2 tablespoons nutritional yeast
½ teaspoon white soy miso (or chickpea miso)

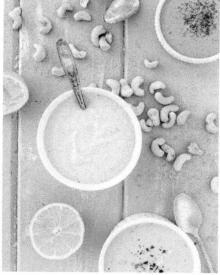

Combine the cashews, ¼ cup of the reserved soaking water, the lemon juice, nutritional yeast, and miso in a food processor or blender and process until smooth. Add up to 2 tablespoons more water for a thinner sauce. Store in an airtight container in the refrigerator for up to 7 days. The cheese will thicken when chilled, so you may need to add more water to thin it back out (unless you want a cheese spread, as described in the Variations).

VARIATIONS

▷ Smoked Gouda Cheese Sauce: Add 1 teaspoon smoked paprika, ½ teaspoon garlic powder, and ½ teaspoon dried dill.

▷ Pepperjack Cheese Sauce: Add ½ teaspoon onion powder, ½ teaspoon garlic powder, and 1 teaspoon red pepper flakes.

▷ Mixed Herb Cheese Sauce: Add 2 teaspoons dried mixed herbs of your choice. I prefer ½ teaspoon dried thyme, ½ teaspoon dried parsley, ½ teaspoon dried oregano, and ½ teaspoon dried basil, but any blend will do.

▷ Melty Cheese: For cheese that seems melty and browns when baked—for the main recipe or any of the variations—increase the water to ⅔ cup and add 1 tablespoon arrowroot powder or cornstarch. Transfer the cheese to a small pot and heat over medium heat, stirring constantly, 3 to 4 minutes, until it's thickened but still drips slowly off a spoon. Pour it on top of whatever you're baking and proceed with that recipe's instructions.

▷ Cheese Spread: Use only 3 tablespoons water, or use the regular amount and chill the cheese sauce for at least 24 hours. The sauce will thicken into a spread.

17

Pepita Parmesan

MAKES 3 CUPS

PREP TIME: **5** minutes
ACTIVE TIME: **2 minutes**

2½ cups pepitas (pumpkin seeds)
½ cup nutritional yeast
1½ teaspoons lemon juice

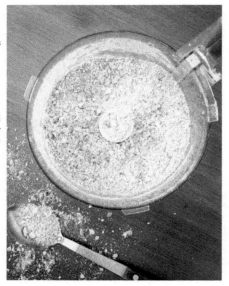

Combine all of the ingredients in a food processor and pulse until broken down into a coarse powder. Transfer to an airtight container. Leftovers will keep in the fridge for up to 2 weeks.

Pickled Red Cabbage & Onion Relish

MAKES 5 CUPS

PREP TIME: **10 minutes**
ACTIVE TIME: **10 minutes**
INACTIVE TIME: **3 to 4 hours**

2 cups apple cider vinegar, plus more if needed
⅔ cup brown sugar (or coconut sugar)
1 teaspoon salt
3 allspice berries
3 cloves
1 medium red onion, halved and very thinly sliced
3 cups shredded or very thinly sliced red cabbage

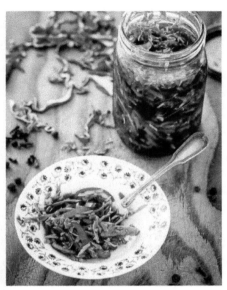

1. Combine the vinegar, sugar, salt, allspice, and cloves in a small pot and bring to a boil. Once the sugar has completely dissolved, after about 1 minute, remove from the heat and set aside.

2. Pack the onion and cabbage in a large pickling jar or an airtight container. Pour the vinegar mixture over the vegetables. If the vegetables are not completely submerged, add more vinegar until they are. Seal the container and shake to fully combine. Refrigerate for 3 to 4 hours before using. Leftovers will keep in the fridge for 7 to 10 days.

Cream of Mushroom Soup

MAKES 3½ CUPS

PREP	TIME:	**8**	**minutes**
ACTIVE	TIME:	**20**	**minutes**
INACTIVE TIME: **30 minutes**			

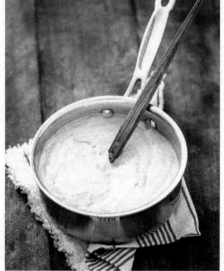

½ large (1½- to 2 lb) head cauliflower, broken into florets
2 teaspoons vegan butter (soy-free if necessary)
8 ounces cremini mushrooms (or button mushrooms), sliced
2 teaspoons liquid aminos (or gluten-free tamari; use coconut aminos to be soy-free)
½ cup raw cashews (if you don't have a high-speed blender, soak in warm water for at least 30 minutes and drain; discard the water)
1 cup unsweetened nondairy milk (soy-free if necessary)
2 tablespoons nutritional yeast
1 tablespoon arrowroot powder (or cornstarch)
1 teaspoon dried thyme
½ teaspoon garlic powder
½ teaspoon salt

1. Place the cauliflower in a steamer basket over a pot of boiling water and cover. Steam the cauliflower until tender, 7 to 10 minutes.

2. Meanwhile, melt the butter in a large frying pan over medium heat. Add the mushrooms and liquid aminos and cook until tender, about 8 minutes. Remove from the heat.

3. Combine the steamed cauliflower, cashews, milk, nutritional yeast, arrowroot powder, thyme, garlic powder, and salt in a blender and blend until smooth. Add the mushrooms (and if desired, their cooking liquid) and pulse until they're in small bits incorporated throughout. You can use the soup right away in a recipe.

4. If you are not using it right away, let it cool completely before transferring to an airtight container. The soup will keep for 5 to 7 days in the fridge or 2 months in the freezer. If you freeze it, let it thaw completely before using.

VARIATION

▷ Turn this into the type of soup you eat in a bowl (novel idea, I know, but settle down, casserole lover): Combine the soup with 2 cups water or low-sodium vegetable broth in a pot and heat over medium heat, stirring occasionally, until heated through.

Avocado Ranch Dressing

MAKES 1¾ CUPS

PREP TIME: **5 minutes**
ACTIVE TIME: **5 minutes**

1 avocado, pitted and peeled
1 cup unsweetened nondairy milk (nut-free and/or soy-free
if necessary)
2 tablespoons lemon juice
1 tablespoon apple cider vinegar
1 teaspoon agave syrup
½ teaspoon garlic powder
½ teaspoon onion powder
½ teaspoon dried oregano
½ teaspoon salt
¼ teaspoon celery seed

¼ teaspoon dried dill

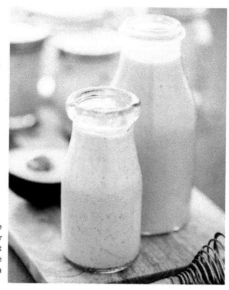

In a food processor or blender, combine all of the
ingredients. Process until smooth. For a thinner
dressing, you can add more nondairy milk until it
reaches your desired consistency. Refrigerate the
dressing until ready to use. Leftovers will keep in an
airtight container in the fridge for 1 to 2 days.

Lemon Tahini Sauce

MAKES 1 CUP

PREP TIME: **5 minutes**
ACTIVE TIME: **5 minutes**

½ cup tahini (gluten-free if necessary)
¼ cup unsweetened nondairy milk (nut-free and/or soy-free if necessary)
3 tablespoons lemon juice
2 tablespoons maple syrup
1 tablespoon liquid aminos (or gluten-free tamari; use coconut aminos to be soy-free)
½ teaspoon ground ginger
¼ teaspoon garlic powder

Combine all of the ingredients in a cup or small bowl and stir with a fork until combined and smooth. Chill until ready to use. The sauce will thicken the longer it chills, so you may need to add water to thin it out before using it. Refrigerate in an airtight container for up to 7 days.

VEGAN BREAKFAST

VEGAN DISHES TO GET EVERYONE'S DAY OFF TO A GOOD START

Tofu Rancheros

SERVES 4 OR 5

PREP TIME: **10 minutes** (not including time to make 15-Minute Refried Beans)
ACTIVE TIME: **20 minutes**

scrambled tofu
1 teaspoon olive oil
½ medium yellow onion, diced
One 14-ounce block extra firm tofu
2 tablespoons vegetable broth, plus more if needed
1 teaspoon black salt (kala namak; or regular salt)
1 teaspoon ground cumin
½ teaspoon paprika
¼ teaspoon ground turmeric
3 tablespoons nutritional yeast, optional
1 tablespoon lemon juice
Black pepper to taste

rancheros

8 to 10 corn tortillas (2 per person)

½ batch 15-Minute Refried Beans

Salsa
Chopped fresh cilantro
Sliced avocado, optional
Shredded cabbage or lettuce, optional
Sliced radishes, optional
Chopped green onions, optional
Lime wedges

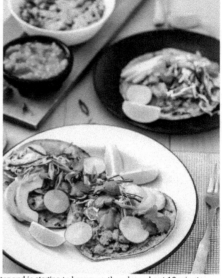

1. **To make the scrambled tofu:** Heat the olive oil in a large skillet over medium heat. Add the onion and sauté for 3-4 minutes. Crumble the tofu into the pan. Cook, stirring gently, until the tofu is no longer releasing any water and is starting to brown on the edges, about 10 minutes. Meanwhile, combine broth, black salt, cumin, paprika, and turmeric in a small cup.

2. Once the tofu has stopped releasing water, add the broth mixture. Cook for about 5 minutes more, until the liquid is absorbed. If it begins to stick, add another tablespoon of broth to deglaze the pan and reduce the heat. Add the nutritional yeast (if using) and lemon juice and cook for about 1 minute more. Remove from the heat and cover the pan to keep warm.

3. **To make the rancheros:** Heat a small pan over medium heat. Place a tortilla in the pan and cook for about 1 minute, flip it, and cook for about 30 seconds more. Transfer to a plate and cover with aluminum foil. Repeat with the remaining tortillas.

4. Spread some refried beans over each tortilla. Top with tofu scramble, a little salsa, and cilantro. If desired, you can also top with avocado slices, shredded cabbage, radish slices, and/or green onions. Serve immediately with a lime wedge. Any leftover scramble can be kept in an airtight container in the fridge for 3 to 4 days.

Maple–Peanut Butter Pancakes

MAKES 8 PANCAKES

PREP TIME: **10 minutes**
ACTIVE TIME: **25 minutes**

¾ cup oat flour (certified gluten-free)
¾ cup gluten-free flour blend (soy-free if necessary)
1 tablespoon cornstarch
1 tablespoon baking powder
½ teaspoon salt
1¼ cups nondairy milk (nut-free and/or soy-free if necessary)
1½ cup maple syrup, plus more for serving
¼ cup unsalted, unsweetened peanut butter (or nut or seed butter of your choice)
1 tablespoon apple cider vinegar
1 teaspoon vanilla extract
Vegan cooking spray (soy-free if necessary)
Vegan butter (soy-free if necessary), optional

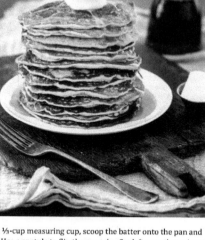

1. If you're not serving the pancakes immediately, see Tip below. In a large bowl, whisk together the oat flour, gluten-free flour, cornstarch, baking powder, and salt. In a medium bowl, whisk together the milk, maple syrup, peanut butter, vinegar, and vanilla. Add the wet ingredients to the dry and stir until combined.

2. Heat a large frying pan or griddle over medium heat for a couple of minutes. Lightly spray with cooking spray. Using a ⅓-cup measuring cup, scoop the batter onto the pan and cook until the top begins to bubble and the edges begin to lift. Use a spatula to flip the pancake. Cook for another minute or two. Gently lift the edge of the pancake to make sure it's golden brown, then transfer the pancake to a plate (or the oven, as in Tip below). Repeat with the remaining batter, taking care to regrease the pan between pancakes.

3. Serve the pancakes topped with a bit of butter (if desired) and a drizzle of maple syrup. Keep leftovers in an airtight container in the fridge for 1 to 2 days.

VARIATIONS

▷ These can also be made by replacing the oat flour, gluten-free flour, and cornstarch with 1½ cups unbleached all-purpose flour. If the batter is too thick, you may need to add a few tablespoons of nondairy milk to thin it out.

▷ You can also use this batter to make waffles by cooking it in a waffle maker according to the machine instructions.

TIP

▷ If you're not planning to serve the pancakes right away, preheat the oven to its lowest setting before you start preparing your batter. Place a cooling rack on a baking sheet. Once a pancake is done, transfer it to the cooling rack and place the sheet in the oven. Continue transferring all pancakes to the rack (avoiding overlapping if possible) and keep them there for up to 20 minutes.

Savory Breakfast Casserole

SERVES 10 TO 12

PREP TIME: **10 minutes** (not including time to make Quick Bacon Crumbles)
ACTIVE TIME: **20 minutes**
INACTIVE TIME: **40 to 45 minutes**

Olive oil spray
One 14-ounce block extra firm tofu
3 cups unsweetened nondairy milk (nut-free if necessary)
2½ cups chickpea flour
2 tablespoons lemon juice
2 tablespoons nutritional yeast
1½ teaspoons black salt (kala namak; or regular salt)
1½ teaspoons garlic powder
1 teaspoon mustard powder
¾ teaspoon ground turmeric
Black pepper to taste
1 teaspoon olive oil
½ medium yellow onion, diced
1 red bell pepper, diced
One 16-ounce bag frozen hash browns
Quick Bacon Crumbles
4 green onions, chopped (green and white parts)

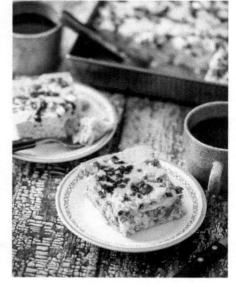

1. Preheat the oven to 400°F. Lightly spray a 9 × 13-inch baking dish with olive oil.

2. Gently squeeze the tofu over the sink, releasing any extra water. Add the tofu, milk, chickpea flour, lemon juice, nutritional yeast, salt, garlic powder, mustard powder, turmeric, and pepper to a blender and blend until smooth. Pour into your largest bowl.

3. Heat the olive oil in a large frying pan over medium heat. Add the onion and bell pepper and sauté until just barely tender. Pour them into the bowl and return the pan to the stove. Add the hash browns to the pan and cook for about 5 minutes, stirring occasionally, until thawed and golden in color. Remove from the heat and pour into the bowl.

4. Add the bacon crumbles to the bowl and stir until combined. Pour into the prepared baking dish and sprinkle the green onions over the top. Bake for 35 minutes, or until firm and a toothpick inserted in the center comes out clean. Remove from the oven and let rest for 5 to 10 minutes before serving. Leftovers will keep in an airtight container in the fridge for 4 to 5 days.

Everyone's Favorite Oatmeal

SERVES 1

PREP TIME: **2 minutes**
ACTIVE TIME: **8 minutes**

1½ cups water
1 cup rolled oats (certified gluten-free if necessary; see Tip)
¼ cup nondairy milk (nut-free and/or soy-free if necessary)
1 to 2 tablespoons maple syrup
1 teaspoon ground cinnamon
Salt to taste

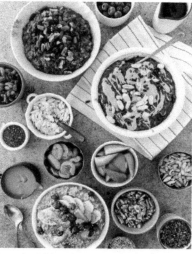

1. Combine the water and oats in a small saucepan or pot and bring to a boil. Reduce to a simmer and cook, untouched, for 3 to 4 minutes, until slightly thick and sticky.

2. Add the milk, maple syrup, cinnamon, and salt and cook for 1 to 2 minutes more, until it's heated through and has reached your desired thickness. Remove from the heat and transfer to a serving bowl. Serve immediately with your choice of toppings.

VARIATIONS

▷ Simple Fruit and Nut Oatmeal: Once cooked, top oatmeal with ⅓ cup fresh fruit (sliced banana, chopped strawberries, sliced nectarine or peach, blueberries, raspberries, blackberries) and/or 2 tablespoons chopped dried fruit 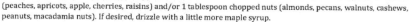 (peaches, apricots, apple, cherries, raisins) and/or 1 tablespoon chopped nuts (almonds, pecans, walnuts, cashews, peanuts, macadamia nuts). If desired, drizzle with a little more maple syrup.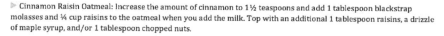

▷ Cinnamon Raisin Oatmeal: Increase the amount of cinnamon to 1½ teaspoons and add 1 tablespoon blackstrap molasses and ¼ cup raisins to the oatmeal when you add the milk. Top with an additional 1 tablespoon raisins, a drizzle of maple syrup, and/or 1 tablespoon chopped nuts.

▷ Peanut Butter and Banana Oatmeal: When adding the milk, add ½ cup sliced bananas and 1 tablespoon peanut butter. Top with a few more banana slices, 1 tablespoon chopped peanuts, and drizzles of peanut butter and maple syrup. You could also add a couple of tablespoons of chocolate chips to take it over the top.

▷ Double Chocolate Oatmeal: Stir in 2 tablespoons cocoa powder when you add the milk. After removing from the heat, stir in 1 to 2 tablespoons chocolate chips. Top with chopped nuts and/or cacao nibs.

▷ Fruit Pie Oatmeal: Add ⅓ cup chopped fruit of your choice (apple, pear, strawberries, bananas, blueberries, blackberries, cherries, peach, pear, persimmon) to the pot when adding the oats. Top with ¼ cup of the same fruit and/or 1 tablespoon chopped nuts.

Vanilla French Toast with Strawberry Sauce

SERVES 4

PREP TIME: **15 minutes** (not including time to make Vanilla Whipped Cream)
ACTIVE TIME: **35 minutes**

French toast
1 vanilla bean
1 cup plain or vanilla nondairy milk (nut-free and/or soy-free if necessary)
½ cup canned coconut milk (or vegan creamer)
½ cup chickpea flour
2 tablespoons maple syrup
1½ tablespoons arrowroot powder
1 teaspoon vanilla extract
¼ teaspoon salt
Vegan cooking spray (soy-free if necessary)
8 vegan bread slices (the thicker the better; gluten-free if necessary)
Vanilla Whipped Cream, optional

Powdered sugar (or xylitol) for dusting, optional
Sliced almonds, optional

strawberry sauce
4 cups chopped strawberries (fresh or frozen)
1 tablespoon cornstarch
1 to 2 tablespoons agave syrup (or maple syrup; depending on sweetness preference)
1 tablespoon lemon juice
1 tablespoon water

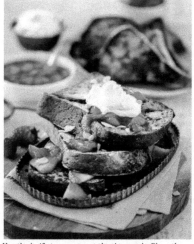

1. Use a paring knife to make a slit lengthwise down the side of the vanilla bean. You don't want to cut it in half—just split it open. Use the knife to scrape out the tiny seeds. Place the seeds in a large shallow bowl or baking dish.

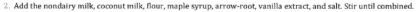

2. Add the nondairy milk, coconut milk, flour, maple syrup, arrow-root, vanilla extract, and salt. Stir until combined.

3. Preheat the oven to its lowest setting. Place a cooling rack on a baking sheet. Set aside.

4. Heat a large frying pan or griddle over medium heat for a couple of minutes. Spray the pan generously with cooking spray. Dip 1 or 2 slices of bread (depending on how many will fit in your pan) in the milk mixture and soak for 10 to 15 seconds on each side. Place the slices in the pan and cook until golden and crispy, 3 to 4 minutes on each side. Transfer to the cooling rack and place the baking sheet in the oven to keep warm until ready to serve. Repeat with the remaining slices of bread, respraying the pan each time before adding new slices.

5. **To make the strawberry sauce:** Combine the sauce ingredients in a small pot and bring to a boil. Reduce the heat and simmer, stirring frequently, for 3 to 5 minutes, until thickened. Remove from the heat and keep warm.

6. If you want, slice the pieces of toast in half diagonally before serving. To serve, place two slices of bread (or four halves) on a plate, topped with a dollop of vanilla whipped cream (if using), a scoop of strawberry sauce, and if you desire, a light dusting of powdered sugar. Sprinkle with a few sliced almonds and serve.

Mushroom-Kale Skillet Hash

SERVES 4

PREP TIME: **10 minutes**
ACTIVE TIME: **20 minutes**

2 teaspoons olive oil
½ medium red onion, diced
2 garlic cloves, minced
3 or 4 red potatoes (about 18 ounces, chopped into ½-inch cubes
8 ounces cremini mushrooms, sliced
1½ teaspoons Old Bay Seasoning
Low-sodium vegetable broth, optional
1 bunch (12 to 16 ounces dino kale (aka lacinato or black kale), stems removed, chopped
Salt and black pepper to taste

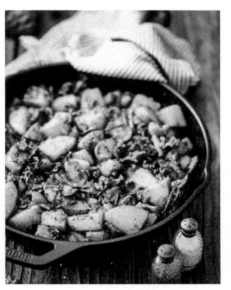

1. Heat the olive oil in a large frying pan, preferably cast iron, over medium heat for a minute. Add the onions and sauté just until translucent.

2. Add the garlic, potatoes, mushrooms, and Old Bay and cook, stirring occasionally, until the mushrooms and potatoes are tender and the potatoes are golden, 15 to 20 minutes. If sticking occurs, add a splash of vegetable broth and lower the heat.

3. Once the veggies are tender, add the kale and cook until wilted. Add salt and pepper and remove from the heat. Serve immediately. Leftovers will keep in an airtight container in the fridge for 2 to 3 days.

Quick & Easy Avocado Toast

SERVES 1

PREP TIME: **3 minutes**
ACTIVE TIME: **5 minutes**

2 vegan bread slices (gluten-free if necessary)
½ avocado, pitted
¾ teaspoon nutritional yeast, optional
1 teaspoon hemp seeds (or sunflower seeds, or toasted pepitas/pumpkin seeds)

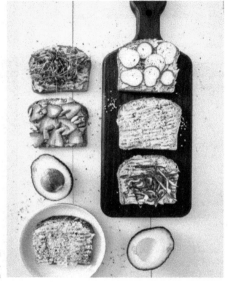

Toast the bread. Scoop half of the avocado onto each slice and use a fork to mash and spread it on the toast. Sprinkle with nutritional yeast (if using) and top with seeds. Serve immediately.

TIP

▶ Ripe avocados work best here. The avocado should be slightly soft but not mushy. If you remove the stem at the top of the avocado, the flesh underneath should be yellow. Green will mean that it's not ripe enough and brown means that it's too ripe (though you could probably still get away with an overripe avocado here).

▶ If you have some leftover Lemon Tahini Sauce, it's magical drizzled on this toast.

EASY VEGAN WEEKNIGHTS

EASY VEGAN WEEKNIGHT MEAL SOLUTIONS

IN THIS CHAPTER

Mexican Pizza with 15-Minute Refried Beans

MAKES 4 PIZZAS, WITH EXTRA BEANS

PREP TIME: **15** (not including time to make Pepperjack Cheese Sauce)
ACTIVE TIME: **25**

15-minute refried beans
1 teaspoon olive oil
1 medium yellow onion, chopped
3 15-ounce cans pinto beans, rinsed and drained
2 tablespoons liquid aminos (or gluten-free tamari; use coconut aminos to be soy-free)
2 teaspoons ground cumin
2 teaspoons ancho chile powder
1½ teaspoons ground coriander
¾ teaspoon smoked paprika
½ cup low-sodium vegetable broth
3 tablespoons canned diced green chiles
2 tablespoons lime juice
Salt and black pepper to taste

pizzas
4 flour tortillas (rice flour or corn tortillas to make them gluten-free; if using corn tortillas, use 2 per person)

Pepperjack Cheese Sauce

1 cup chopped fresh tomatoes
½ cup sliced pitted black olives, optional

Optional toppings: sliced avocado, chopped or shredded greens of your choice, chopped green onions, Pickled Red Cabbage & Onion Relish

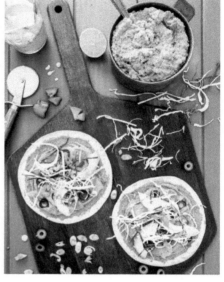

1. Preheat the oven to 400°F. Line one or two baking sheets with aluminum foil or silicone baking mats. Set aside.

2. **To make the refried beans:** Heat the olive oil in a large shallow saucepan over medium heat. Add the onion and sauté until just translucent, 3 to 4 minutes. Add the beans, liquid aminos, cumin, chile powder, coriander, paprika, and broth. Cook for about 5 minutes, until heated through and about half of the liquid has been absorbed.

3. Add the green chiles and lime juice and remove from the heat. Transfer to a food processor and pulse until the beans are mostly smooth with some chunks. Add salt and pepper.

4. **To make the pizzas:** Spread out the tortillas on the baking sheets. Spread refried beans generously over each one. Drizzle the cheese sauce over the beans and sprinkle the chopped tomatoes and olives (if using) over each pizza. Bake for 10 minutes, or until the tortillas are crispy.

5. Top the pizzas with your additional toppings and serve immediately. Leftover beans can be kept in an airtight container in the fridge for 5 to 6 days or frozen for up to 2 months. When reheating, you may need to add a few tablespoons of broth or water to thin them out again.

Potato Leek Soup

SERVES 4 TO 6

PREP TIME: **15 minutes** (not including time to make Quick Bacon Crumbles)
ACTIVE TIME: **25 minutes**
INACTIVE TIME: **15 minutes**

1 teaspoon olive oil
2 leeks, thinly sliced (white and light green parts)
1 garlic clove, minced
2 pounds Yukon gold potatoes, chopped
2 teaspoons dried rosemary
2 teaspoons dried thyme
1 teaspoon ground sage
3 cups low-sodium vegetable broth
2 cups water
1 tablespoon nutritional yeast, optional
1 tablespoon lemon juice
1 teaspoon liquid smoke
Salt and black pepper to taste
Quick Bacon Crumbles, optional
Chopped green onions, optional

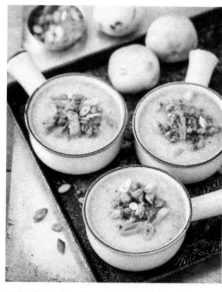

1. In a large pot, heat the olive oil over medium heat. Add the leeks and sauté until soft, about 4 minutes. Add the garlic and sauté for another minute. Add the potatoes, rosemary, thyme, sage, broth, and water. Bring to a boil, then reduce the heat and simmer until the potatoes are tender, about 15 minutes. Turn off the heat.

2. Add the nutritional yeast, lemon juice, and liquid smoke. Use an immersion blender to blend the soup until smooth (or mostly smooth with a few potato chunks—your call). Alternatively, you can transfer the soup in batches to a blender and carefully blend until smooth.

3. Add salt and pepper. Serve topped with bacon crumbles and green onions, if desired. Leftovers will keep in an airtight container in the fridge for 5 to 6 days.

Quick Cauliflower Curry

PREP TIME: **20 minutes**
ACTIVE TIME: **15 minutes**
INACTIVE TIME: **10 minutes**

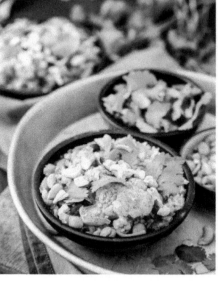

1 tablespoon coconut oil
1 medium yellow onion, diced
2 garlic cloves, minced
1 tablespoon grated fresh ginger
1 tablespoon curry powder
2 teaspoons garam masala
1 teaspoon ground coriander
1 teaspoon ground cumin
½ teaspoon ground turmeric
1 medium (1-pound head cauliflower, broken into florets
8 ounces cremini mushrooms (or button mushrooms), sliced
One 15-ounce can chickpeas, rinsed and drained
One 15-ounce can no-salt-added fire-roasted diced tomatoes
3 cups low-sodium vegetable broth
1 cup plain coconut yogurt (preferably unsweetened)
Salt and black pepper to taste
Chopped fresh cilantro, optional
Chopped cashews, optional (see Variation)
Cooked rice (or vegan bread)

1. Heat the coconut oil in a large pot or Dutch oven over medium heat. Add the onion, garlic, and ginger and sauté until the onion is just becoming translucent. Add the curry powder, garam masala, coriander, cumin, and turmeric and cook until fragrant, about 1 minute.

2. Add the cauliflower, mushrooms, chickpeas, tomatoes and their liquid, and the broth and bring to a boil. Reduce the heat to a simmer and cover. Cook for about 10 minutes, then remove the lid and cook for about 5 minutes more. Stir in the yogurt and cook for a few minutes, until heated through. Add salt and pepper and remove from the heat.

3. Top with chopped cilantro and/or cashews, if desired, and serve with rice or bread. Store leftovers in an airtight container in the fridge for 4 to 5 days.

VARIATION

▶ To make this nut-free, switch out the cashews with pepitas (pumpkin seeds) or sesame seeds.

BBQ Chickpea Salad

SERVES 2 TO 4

PREP TIME: **20 minutes** (not including time to make Avocado Ranch Dressing and Pickled Red Cabbage & Onion Relish)
ACTIVE TIME: **15 minutes**

3 cups cooked chickpeas (or two 15-ounce, rinsed and drained)
2 tablespoons liquid aminos (use coconut aminos to be soy-free)
⅔ cup vegan barbecue sauce (homemade or store-bought)
1 large head romaine lettuce, chopped
1 cup shredded red cabbage
1 cup halved cherry tomatoes
1 cup sliced nectarines (or sliced peaches or chopped mango)
½ cup grated carrot
Avocado Ranch Dressing

Toasted pepitas (pumpkin seeds)
Pickled Red Cabbage & Onion Relish

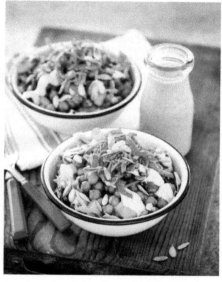

1. Heat a large shallow saucepan over medium heat. Add the chick-peas and liquid aminos and cook, stirring a couple of times, until the liquid has been absorbed, 2 to 3 minutes.

2. Add ⅓ cup of the barbecue sauce and toss to coat. Cook until the sauce has thickened and caramelized, and all the liquid has been absorbed. Add the remaining barbecue sauce and cook until the sauce has thickened and caramelized again. Remove from the heat.

3. In a large bowl, toss together the lettuce, red cabbage, cherry tomatoes, nectarine slices, and carrots. Divide the salad among four bowls and top with the chickpeas. Top with dressing, a sprinkling of the pepitas, and a scoop of the relish. Serve immediately. Leftover beans will keep in an airtight container in the fridge for 3 to 4 days.

Spicy Sesame Soba Noodle Bowl

SERVES 4 TO 6

PREP TIME: **15 minutes**
ACTIVE TIME: **30 minutes**

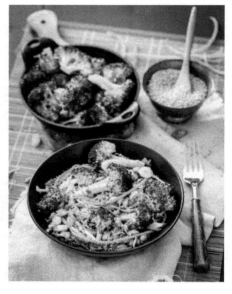

1 bunch broccoli, chopped into florets
2 tablespoons sesame oil
Salt and pepper to taste
¾ cup tahini (gluten-free if necessary)
3 tablespoons tamari (gluten-free if necessary)
2 tablespoons brown rice vinegar
1 to 2 tablespoons sriracha (or other hot sauce)
1 tablespoon maple syrup
1 teaspoon ground ginger
½ teaspoon garlic powder
One 12-ounce package buckwheat soba noodles (or vegan angel hair pasta or spaghetti; gluten-free if necessary)
1½ cups frozen shelled edamame
2 large carrots, peeled and julienned
Sesame seeds
Chopped green onions (green and white parts)

1. Preheat the oven to 425°F. Line a baking sheet with parchment paper or a silicone baking mat. Spread out the broccoli on the sheet and drizzle with the sesame oil, then add salt and pepper. Toss to fully coat. Bake for 15 to 20 minutes, until tender with slightly crispy edges, tossing once halfway through. Remove from the oven and set aside.

2. While the broccoli is roasting, fill a large pot with water and bring to a boil.

3. While you're waiting for the water to boil, you can make the sauce: Combine the tahini, tamari, vinegar, sriracha, maple syrup, ginger, and garlic powder in a medium bowl and stir until combined and smooth. Set aside.

4. Once the water is boiling, add the noodles and cook according to the package instructions until al dente. About 1 minute after you add the noodles to the water, add the edamame. Once the noodles are done, drain and rinse the noodles and edamame with cold water, then drain again. Transfer to a large serving bowl. Stir in the sauce. Add the carrots and roasted broccoli and stir to combine. Serve topped with sesame seeds and green onions. Leftovers will keep in an airtight container in the fridge for 1 to 2 days.

Cheesy Quinoa & Veggies

SERVES 4 TO 6

PREP TIME: **20 minutes** (not including time to make Pepita Parmesan)
ACTIVE TIME: **30 minutes**

1 cup quinoa, thoroughly rinsed
2 cups water
1 teaspoon olive oil
½ medium yellow onion, diced
½ medium (1-pound head cauliflower, broken into small florets
8 ounces fresh green beans, trimmed
2 tablespoons low-sodium vegetable broth (or water)
8 ounces cremini mushrooms (or button mushrooms), sliced
2 medium zucchini, halved lengthwise and sliced
3 tablespoons liquid aminos (or gluten-free tamari; use coconut aminos to be soy-free)
1 teaspoon dried thyme
1 teaspoon dried parsley
1 teaspoon garlic powder
1½ cups cooked great Northern beans (or one 15-ounce can, rinsed and drained)
⅓ cup nutritional yeast
3 cups packed chopped greens (spinach, chard, kale, or collards)
¼ cup lemon juice
Salt and black pepper to taste
Pepita Parmesan, optional

1. Combine the quinoa with the water in a medium pot. Cover and bring to a boil, then reduce the heat and simmer for about 15 minutes, until all the water has been absorbed. Remove from the heat, keeping it covered, and let it rest for about 10 minutes before fluffing with a fork.

2. While the quinoa is cooking, heat the olive oil in a large, shallow saucepan over medium heat. Add the onion and sauté for 2 to 3 minutes. Add the cauliflower, green beans, and broth, cover the pan, and cook for 3 to 4 minutes. Add the mushrooms, zucchini, liquid aminos, thyme, parsley, and garlic powder. Cover and cook, stirring occasionally, until all of the vegetables are tender but not too soft (they should still have a "bite" to them), 6 to 7 minutes. Add the cooked quinoa and the beans, stir, and cook until heated through, about 2 minutes. Stir in the nutritional yeast. Stir in the greens and cook until just beginning to wilt. Add the lemon juice, salt, and pepper and remove from the heat.

3. Serve immediately, topped with Pepita Parmesan (if using). Store any leftovers in an airtight container in the fridge for 3 to 4 days.

Jackfruit Crabless Cakes with Lemon Dill Aïoli

SERVES 3 OR 4

PREP TIME: **15 minutes** (not including time to cook brown rice)
ACTIVE TIME: **20 minutes**

One 20-ounce can jackfruit, thoroughly rinsed and drained
1½ cups cooked cannellini beans/15 oz can, rinsed & drained
4 green onions, finely chopped, plus more for garnish
1 cup cooked brown rice
2 tablespoons chickpea flour, plus more if needed
1 tablespoon vegan mayonnaise (soy-free if necessary)
1 tablespoon Old Bay Seasoning
2 teaspoons liquid aminos (or gluten-free tamari; use coconut aminos to be soy-free)
1 teaspoon dried parsley
½ teaspoon kelp granules
½ teaspoon garlic powder
Salt and black pepper to taste
Sunflower oil (or canola oil) for frying

lemon dill aïoli
¾ cup vegan mayonnaise (soy-free if necessary)
3 tablespoons lemon juice
1½ teaspoons dried dill
¼ teaspoon garlic powder
Salt to taste

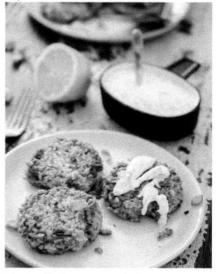

1. Line a baking sheet with parchment paper or a silicone baking mat.

2. Place the jackfruit in a food processor and pulse about five times, until broken up into smaller pieces.

3. Pour the beans into a bowl and use a potato masher to mash them until creamy but still chunky. Add the jackfruit, green onions, brown rice, chickpea flour, mayonnaise, Old Bay, liquid aminos, parsley, kelp granules, garlic powder, salt, and pepper and stir together until combined. The mixture should hold together when you squeeze it. If it doesn't, add chickpea flour by the tablespoon until it does.

4. Scoop up ⅓ cup of the mixture and use your hands to shape it into a patty. Place the patty on the baking sheet. Repeat with the remaining mixture. You should have about 12 patties.

5. Heat a large frying pan, preferably cast iron, over medium heat. Pour in enough oil to coat the bottom and heat for 2 to 3 minutes. Line a plate with paper towels. Place three or four patties in the pan and cook for 3 to 4 minutes on each side, until crispy and browned all over. Place the cooked patties on the plate and top with more paper towels to absorb any excess oil. Repeat with the remaining patties, adding more oil as necessary, until all are cooked.

6. While the cakes are cooking, **make the aïoli:** Combine all the ingredients in a cup and stir together. Chill until ready to use.

7. Garnish the cakes with chopped green onions and serve with the aïoli on the side. Leftovers will keep in an airtight container in the fridge for 3 to 4 days.

KID FRIENDLY VEGAN

VEGAN MEALS THAT KIDS WILL LOVE.

Hidden Veggie Mac 'n' Cheese

SERVES 8

PREP TIME: **15 minutes** (not including time make Pepita Parmesan)
ACTIVE TIME: **30 minutes**

½ medium (1-pound) head cauliflower, broken into florets
2 large carrots, peeled and chopped
½ cup diced radishes
1 pound elbow macaroni (gluten-free if necessary)
1 cup cooked great Northern beans
1 cup unsweetened nondairy milk (nut-free and/or soy-free if necessary)
¾ cup nutritional yeast
¼ cup lemon juice
2 tablespoons no-salt-added tomato paste
2 tablespoons vegan butter (soy-free if necessary), melted
2 teaspoons white soy miso (or chickpea miso)
1 teaspoon onion powder
1 teaspoon garlic powder
½ teaspoon paprika
¼ teaspoon mustard powder
Salt and black pepper to taste
 Pepita Parmesan, optional

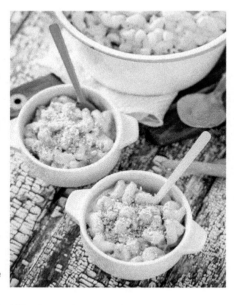

1. Place the cauliflower, carrots, and radishes in a medium pot and cover with water. Bring to a boil and cook the vegetables until easily pierced with a fork, 8 to 10 minutes. Remove from the heat and drain. Set aside.

2. Fill a large pot with water and bring to a boil. Once boiling, add the pasta and cook according to the package instructions until al dente. Remove from the heat, drain well, and return the pasta to the pot.

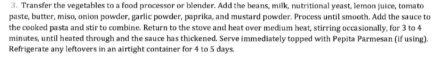

3. Transfer the vegetables to a food processor or blender. Add the beans, milk, nutritional yeast, lemon juice, tomato paste, butter, miso, onion powder, garlic powder, paprika, and mustard powder. Process until smooth. Add the sauce to the cooked pasta and stir to combine. Return to the stove and heat over medium heat, stirring occasionally, for 3 to 4 minutes, until heated through and the sauce has thickened. Serve immediately topped with Pepita Parmesan (if using). Refrigerate any leftovers in an airtight container for 4 to 5 days.

Tempeh Nuggets

MAKES 40 NUGGETS

PREP TIME: **10 minutes**
ACTIVE TIME: **30 minutes**
INACTIVE TIME: **30 minutes**

Two 8-ounce packages tempeh
3 cups low-sodium "no-chicken" flavored vegetable broth (or regular vegetable broth)
2 tablespoons liquid aminos
1 teaspoon dried thyme
1 teaspoon dried marjoram
¾ cup plain vegan yogurt (preferably unsweetened, nut-free if necessary)
¼ cup unsweetened nondairy milk (nut-free if necessary)
3 tablespoons tahini (gluten-free if necessary)
½ teaspoon salt
½ teaspoon onion powder
½ teaspoon garlic powder
¼ teaspoon smoked paprika
1½ cups vegan panko bread crumbs (gluten-free if necessary)
3 tablespoons nutritional yeast
Olive oil spray
Ketchup (or vegan barbecue sauce; homemade or store-bought), for dipping

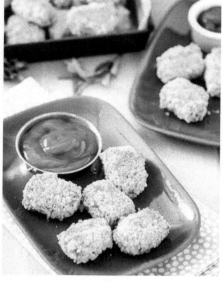

1. Chop each block of tempeh into about 20 chunks, making 40 total nuggets.

2. Combine the broth, liquid aminos, thyme, and marjoram in a large pot. Place the tempeh in the pot and bring to a boil. Once boiling, reduce to a simmer and let the tempeh simmer for about 20 minutes. Remove from the heat and drain (you can save the liquid for another time you need to cook with broth or add a bit of liquid to your pan; it should keep in the fridge for a couple of weeks). Set the tempeh aside to cool until you can handle it.

3. While the tempeh is cooling, combine the yogurt, milk, tahini, salt, onion powder, garlic powder, and paprika in a shallow bowl. In another shallow bowl, combine the bread crumbs and nutritional yeast.

4. Preheat the oven to 375°F. Line a baking sheet with parchment paper or a silicone baking mat.

5. Use one hand to dredge a piece of tempeh in the yogurt mixture and your other hand to toss it in the bread crumbs until fully coated. Place the nugget on the prepared baking sheet. Repeat with the remaining nuggets.

6. Lightly spray the tops of the nuggets with olive oil. Bake for 12 minutes, flip them and spray the tops with olive oil again, and return to the oven for 12 minutes more, or until crispy and golden. Serve immediately with your choice of dipping sauces. Leftovers will keep in an airtight container in the fridge for 3 to 4 days.

Cheesy Trees

SERVES 4, WITH EXTRA SAUCE

PREP TIME: **10 minutes**
ACTIVE TIME: **15 minutes**
INACTIVE TIME: **60 minutes**

1 cup chopped Yukon gold potatoes
½ cup peeled, chopped carrot
1 bunch (1 pound) broccoli chopped into florets
¼ cup raw cashews, soaked in warm water for 1 hour and drained, water reserved
¾ cup reserved soaking water
¼ cup nutritional yeast
2 tablespoons lemon juice
1 tablespoon olive oil
½ teaspoon onion powder
½ teaspoon garlic powder
½ teaspoon salt
Salt and black pepper to taste

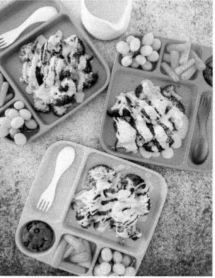

1. Place the potatoes and carrots in a medium pot and cover with water. Bring to a boil and cook for 8 to 10 minutes, until the vegetables are easily pierced with a fork.

2. While you're boiling the potatoes and carrots, place the broccoli in a steamer basket over a pot of boiling water and cover. Steam the broccoli until tender, 8 to 10 minutes. Once tender, remove from the heat but keep warm until ready to serve.

3. Drain the potatoes and carrots and transfer them to the blender. Add the cashews, reserved soaking water, nutritional yeast, lemon juice, olive oil, onion powder, garlic powder, and salt. Blend until completely smooth.

4. Serve the broccoli with a pinch of salt and pepper and a few dollops of cheese sauce. Store any leftover cheese sauce in an airtight container in the fridge for 3 to 4 days.

VARIATION

▶ If your kids don't like broccoli, try using cauliflower or another vegetable they like instead.

PB&J Roll-Ups

MAKES 4 ROLL-UPS, WITH EXTRA SPREAD

PREP TIME: **5 minutes**
ACTIVE TIME: **5 minutes**

1 cup peanut butter (or nut or seed butter of your choice)
Half of a 12-ounce vacuum-packed block extra firm silken tofu
1 tablespoon maple syrup, optional
Salt to taste, optional
4 large flour tortillas (or brown rice tortillas or lavash wraps)
1 pound strawberries, hulled and sliced

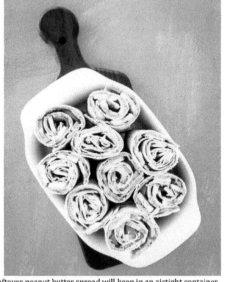

1. Combine the peanut butter, tofu, maple syrup (if using), and salt (if using) in a food processor and process until smooth.

2. Spread 2 to 3 tablespoons of the peanut butter spread on a tortilla. Make a layer of strawberry slices on top of the peanut butter. Roll up the tortilla into a log. Chop into three or four sections. Repeat with the remaining tortillas.

3. Serve immediately. To serve later, wrap each roll-up (all sections) in plastic wrap and refrigerate, if possible (if it's in a lunch box for a few hours, it will be fine). Any leftover peanut butter spread will keep in an airtight container in the fridge for about 7 days.

VARIATION

▷ Replace the strawberries with thinly sliced apples, bananas, or other fruit.

43

Fruity Granola Bars

MAKES 12 BARS

PREP TIME: **5 minutes**
ACTIVE TIME: **10 minutes**
INACTIVE TIME: **80 minutes**

1 cup pitted Medjool dates
½ cup peanut butter (or almond butter or nut or seed butter of your choice)
¼ cup + 2 tablespoons apple juice
¼ cup coconut oil, melted
1 teaspoon vanilla extract
½ teaspoon salt
2½ cups rolled oats (certified gluten-free if necessary)
¾ cup chopped dried fruit (cherries, apricots, raisins, blueberries, apples, peach, and/or mango)
½ cup chopped nuts (almonds, pecans, walnuts, cashews, pistachios, and/or peanuts; see Variation)
½ cup sunflower (or pepitas/pumpkin seeds, or mixture of both)

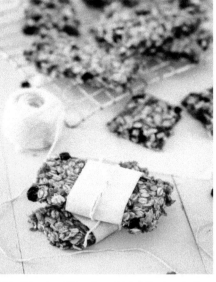

1. Preheat the oven to 300°F. Line a 9 × 13-inch baking dish with parchment paper.

2. Combine the dates, nut butter, apple juice, coconut oil, vanilla, and salt in a food processor and process until smooth. Set aside.

3. In a large bowl, stir together the oats, dried fruit, nuts, and seeds. Add the date mixture and stir until combined. Pour into the prepared baking dish and use a silicone spatula to flatten and smooth it.

4. Bake for 20 minutes, or until lightly golden, then remove from the oven and let cool completely before transferring to the refrigerator to chill for at least 1 hour.

5. Remove from the refrigerator and use the parchment paper to lift the granola out of the baking dish. Slice into 12 bars. Store in an airtight container in the fridge. The bars will keep for 7 to 10 days.

VARIATION

▷ To make these bars nut-free, use a seed butter and replace the nuts with more sunflower and/or pepitas.

Bean & Cheese Quesadillas

MAKES 4 QUESADILLAS

PREP TIME: **15 minutes** (not including time to make 15-Minute Refried Beans and Basic Cashew Cheese Sauce)
ACTIVE TIME: **10 minutes**

2 cups 15-Minute _Refried Beans_
4 flour tortillas (gluten-free if necessary)
Basic Cashew Cheese Sauce
Salsa and/or guacamole

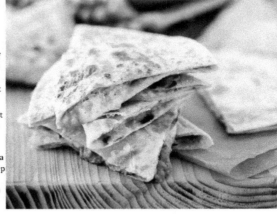

1. Spread ½ cup of the beans on one half of a tortilla. Drizzle cheese sauce over the beans. Gently fold the other side of the tortilla over the beans and cheese. Repeat with the remaining tortillas.

2. Heat a large frying pan, preferably cast iron, over medium-heat. Place one to two (if they'll both fit) quesadillas in the pan and cook for 3 to 4 minutes on each side, until golden and crispy. Transfer them to a plate and cover with aluminum foil to keep warm. Repeat with the remaining quesadillas. Serve immediately with salsa and/or guacamole.

TIP

▷ To make these quesadillas come together in a snap, you can prepare the refried beans and/or the cheese sauce in advance. It's also a great way to use up any leftover refried beans you may have from making Mexican Pizza with _15-Minute Refried Beans_ .

▷ To ensure that this dish is soy-free, remember to use coconut aminos in the refried beans and chickpea miso in the cashew cheese sauce.

VEGAN SNACKS & FINGER FOODS

VEGAN FOOD COOL ENOUGH FOR SPORTS GAMES, SLEEPOVERS, AND JUST HANGING OUT

Make-Your-Own Cheese Pizza

MAKES 1 LARGE PIZZA, WITH EXTRA SAUCE

PREP TIME: **20 minutes** (not including time to make Basic Cashew Cheese Sauce or your own pizza dough)
ACTIVE TIME: **25 minutes**

pizza sauce

One 15-ounce can no-salt-added tomato sauce
One 6-ounce can no-salt-added tomato paste
1 tablespoon extra virgin olive oil
1 teaspoon dried basil
1 teaspoon dried oregano
2 pinches of garlic powder
½ cup water

Salt and black pepper to taste

pizzas

1 or more individual store-bought pizza crusts (or you can use your favorite pizza dough recipe—most are vegan; use gluten-free if necessary)

Basic Cashew Cheese Sauce

Assorted pizza toppings, such as sliced mushrooms, bell peppers, red onion, artichoke hearts, chopped fresh tomatoes, sundried tomatoes, olives, pineapple, chopped fresh basil

Sliced vegan sausage, chopped chickenless strips, or beefless crumbles, optional

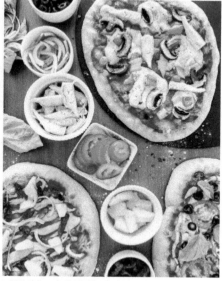

1. **To make the pizza sauce:** Combine the tomato sauce, tomato paste, olive oil, basil, oregano, garlic powder, and water in a medium pot and bring to a boil. Reduce to a simmer and cook, stirring occasionally, for 15 to 20 minutes, until thickened.

2. While the sauce is simmering, follow the instructions for your pizza crust(s) or pizza dough recipe for preheating the oven and preparation. Prepare your toppings and place them on a tray or set them out on the counter, getting them ready for the teens to invade.

3. Once the oven is hot, spread sauce on top of the crust(s), leaving 1 inch around the perimeter. Drizzle or spoon the cheese sauce over the top, using as much or as little as you like. If the crusts are small enough, everyone can add make their own individual pizza. If the crusts are large, you can let each person add toppings of their choice to half of a pizza.

4. Bake the pizza(s) according to the recipe instructions. Once done, remove the pizza(s) from the oven, slice, and serve.

Smashed Lentil Tacos

MAKES 12 TACOS

PREP TIME: **15 minutes** (not including time to make Pepperjack Cheese Sauce)
ACTIVE TIME: **35 minutes**

1 quart low-sodium vegetable broth
2 cups brown lentils, rinsed and picked through
2 teaspoons ancho chile powder
2 teaspoons ground cumin
1½ teaspoons ground coriander
1 teaspoon garlic powder
1 teaspoon onion powder
½ teaspoon smoked paprika
3 tablespoons liquid aminos (or gluten-free tamari; use coconut aminos to be soy-free)
2 tablespoons lime juice
Salt and black pepper to taste
12 corn tortillas
Shredded cabbage
Guacamole or sliced avocado, optional
Salsa, optional
Pepperjack Cheese Sauce, optional

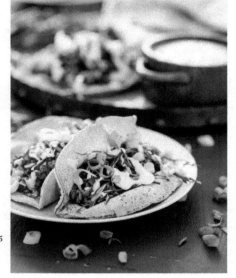

1. In a medium pot, combine the broth, lentils, ancho chile powder, cumin, coriander, garlic powder, onion powder, and paprika. Cover the pot and bring to a boil. Once boiling, crack the lid and reduce the heat to a simmer. Let simmer until the liquid has cooked away, 15 to 20 minutes. Remove from the heat.

2. Add the liquid aminos, lime juice, salt, and pepper. Use a potato masher to smash the lentils until they slightly resemble taco meat.

3. While the lentils are cooking, you can prepare the tortillas. Heat a large frying pan, preferably cast iron, over medium heat. Place a tortilla in the pan and once the edges begin to curl up (after about 30 seconds), flip and cook for another 30 seconds. Place the heated tortilla on a plate and cover with aluminum foil. Repeat with the remaining tortillas.

4. To serve, scoop a bit of the smashed lentils onto a tortilla. Top with cabbage, and add guacamole, salsa, and/or cheese sauce (if using).

Tempeh Sloppy Joe Sliders

SERVES 8

PREP TIME: **5 minutes**
ACTIVE TIME: **20 minutes**

1 teaspoon olive oil
1 medium red onion, diced
1 red bell pepper, diced
2 garlic cloves, minced
Two 8-ounce packages tempeh (soy-free if necessary), crumbled
½ cup low-sodium vegetable broth (or water)
One 15-ounce can no-salt-added crushed tomatoes
One 6-ounce can no-salt-added tomato paste
¼ cup liquid aminos (or gluten-free tamari; use coconut aminos to be soy-free)
2 tablespoons maple syrup
1½ teaspoons ground cumin
1 teaspoon dried parsley
1 teaspoon dried thyme
1 teaspoon smoked paprika
Salt and black pepper to taste
16 slider or 8 full-size vegan burger buns (gluten-free if necessary)
Vegan mayonnaise (soy-free if necessary), optional
Sliced avocado, optional

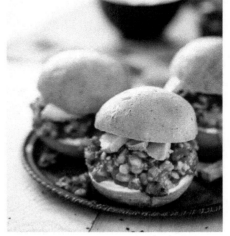

1. Heat the olive oil in a large, shallow saucepan over medium heat. Add the onion and cook until slightly translucent. Add the bell pepper and garlic and cook for a couple of minutes more, until the garlic is fragrant. Add the tempeh, broth, crushed tomatoes, tomato paste, liquid aminos, maple syrup, cumin, parsley, thyme, and paprika. Cook, stirring occasionally, until the tempeh is tender and the sauce is thick, 10 to 12 minutes. Add the salt and pepper, then remove from the heat.

2. Serve on the burger buns, slathered with mayonnaise and topped with avocado (if using).

Tater Totchos

SERVES 6 TO 8

PREP TIME: **10 minutes**
ACTIVE TIME: **30 minutes**

One 32-ounce bag frozen potato tots (most are vegan, but be sure to double-check before buying)

nacho cheese sauce

1 cup chopped Yukon gold potatoes
½ cup peeled, chopped carrot
¾ cup water
¼ cup nutritional yeast
2 tablespoons tahini (gluten-free if necessary)
1½ tablespoons pickled jalapeño juice
1 tablespoon canned diced green chiles
1 tablespoon lime juice
2 teaspoons sunflower oil (or grapeseed oil), optional
1 scant tablespoon minced pickled jalapeño, optional
1 teaspoon ground cumin
½ teaspoon onion powder

beans

1 teaspoon olive oil
1 medium red onion, diced
2 garlic cloves, minced
1 red bell pepper, diced
3 cups cooked black beans (or two 15-ounce cans, rinsed and drained)
¼ cup liquid aminos (or gluten-free tamari; use coconut aminos to be soy-free)
2 teaspoons ground cumin
2 teaspoons ancho chile powder
1 teaspoon ground coriander
½ teaspoon paprika
3 tablespoons canned diced green chiles
Juice of 1 lime
Salt and black pepper to taste

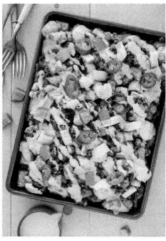

Optional toppings: chopped green onions, chopped fresh tomato, pickled jalapeños, guacamole or chunks of avocado, vegan sour cream

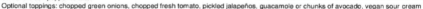
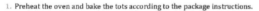
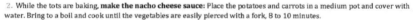

1. Preheat the oven and bake the tots according to the package instructions.

2. While the tots are baking, **make the nacho cheese sauce:** Place the potatoes and carrots in a medium pot and cover with water. Bring to a boil and cook until the vegetables are easily pierced with a fork, 8 to 10 minutes.

3. Drain the vegetables and transfer them to your food processor. Add the water, nutritional yeast, tahini, pickled jalapeño juice, green chiles, lime juice, sunflower oil (if using), pickled jalapeño (if using), cumin, and onion powder. Process until completely smooth. Set aside.

4. **To make the beans:** Heat the olive oil in a large frying pan over medium heat. Add the onions, garlic, and red bell pepper. Sauté until the onions are slightly translucent. Add the beans, liquid aminos, cumin, ancho chile powder, coriander, and paprika. Cook until the liquid has been absorbed and the beans are heated through. Add the green chiles and lime juice and cook until the liquid has been absorbed, about 1 minute. Remove from the heat and add salt and pepper.

5. Spread out the tots on a large platter or small baking sheet. Top with the beans, then drizzle the sauce over the beans. If desired, top with green onions, tomato, jalapeños, guacamole, and/or sour cream. Serve immediately.

Just Fries

MAKES AS MUCH AS YOU WANT

PREP TIME: **10 minutes**
ACTIVE TIME: **10 minutes**
INACTIVE TIME: **25 minutes**

Olive oil spray
1 russet potato per person (or ½ potato per person if using
as a side dish), peeled (see Tip)
Salt and black pepper to taste
Garlic powder, optional
Vegan sauces (such as ketchup, barbecue sauce, mustard,
or ranch dressing; gluten-free, nut-free, and/or soy-free if
necessary), for dipping

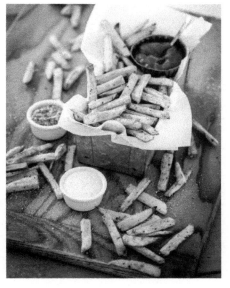

1. Preheat the oven to 450°F . Line baking sheets with
aluminum foil—you can fit about 2 potatoes per baking
sheet, so do the math. Lightly spray the foil with olive oil.

2. Slice each potato into similarly sized strips or
wedges. It's important that they're equal size so that they
cook evenly.

3. Spread out the fries on the prepared baking sheets.
Spray a light coating of olive oil over the fries. Sprinkle
them with salt, pepper, and garlic powder (if using). Toss
to coat and rearrange the slices on the sheet so they're
not touching (as much as possible). This will help them
get more crispy.

4. Bake for 25 to 30 minutes, flipping them once halfway through to ensure even cooking. Once they're crispy and
lightly browned on the outside but easily pierced with a fork, they're ready. Remove from the oven and serve
immediately with the preferred dipping sauce(s).

TIP

▷ You don't need to peel the potatoes if you're in a hurry, but I recommend it—it really makes a difference in flavor and texture.

Hot Fudge Ice Cream Sundaes

SERVES 8

PREP TIME: **15 minutes** (not including time to make Vanilla Whipped Cream)
ACTIVE TIME: **30 minutes** INACTIVE TIME: **6 hours**

vanilla ice cream

1½ cups raw cashews, soaked in warm water for 1 hour and drained, water discarded
One 13.5-ounce can coconut milk
½ cup maple syrup
1 tablespoon arrowroot powder
2 tablespoons grapeseed oil (or sunflower oil)
1½ teaspoons vanilla powder
1 teaspoon vanilla extract
¼ teaspoon salt

hot fudge

½ cup vegan chocolate chips (or chunks)
1 cup lite coconut milk
¼ cup cocoa powder
¼ cup brown sugar (or coconut sugar)
2 tablespoons coconut oil, melted
1 tablespoon arrowroot powder
¼ teaspoon salt

toppings (all optional)

Vanilla Whipped Cream

Chopped nuts (such as almonds, peanuts, pecans)
Chopped fruit (such as strawberries, bananas, mango)
Vegan chocolate chips & sprinkles
Vegan marshmallows (soy-free if necessary)
Crumbled vegan cookies (gluten-free if necessary)
Caramel Cashew Granola (or store-bought vegan granola)
Maraschino cherries

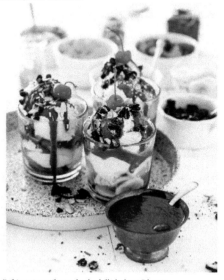

1. **To make the ice cream** : Combine the cashews, coconut milk, maple syrup, arrowroot, oil, vanilla powder, vanilla extract, and salt in a blender and blend until completely smooth. Refrigerate until completely chilled, about 2 hours.

2. Process in your ice cream maker, according to the manufacturer's instructions. When the ice cream reaches the consistency of a thick soft-serve, transfer to a glass or metal bowl. Place a piece of parchment paper on top of the ice cream to prevent contact with air (thus reducing freezer burn), then cover the bowl with plastic wrap. Freeze the ice cream for at least 3 or 4 hours before serving. You may need to let the ice cream soften for about 5 minutes before serving.

3. **To make the hot fudge** : Melt the chocolate in a double boiler or a heatproof bowl on top of a pan of boiling water, stirring frequently, until completely smooth. While the chocolate is melting, whisk together the coconut milk, cocoa powder, sugar, coconut oil, arrow-root, and salt in a medium bowl.

4. Slowly whisk the milk mixture into the melted chocolate and stir until heated through, 1 to 2 minutes. Remove from the heat. If you make this in advance, once it has cooled, you can refrigerate the sauce in an airtight container. It will get very thick, so you will have to reheat it before serving.

5. Prepare all of the toppings you plan on serving. To assemble, scoop as much ice cream as desired into a bowl, drizzle hot fudge all over it, and top with all the preferred toppings.

THE FAVORITES - VEGAN STYLE

VEGAN FOOD FOR YOUR "MEAT AND POTATOES" FAMILY MEMBERS

Cheese-Stuffed Meatballs

SERVES 4

PREP TIME: **15 minutes** (not including time to make Smoked Gouda Cheese Sauce and Sun-Dried Tomato Marinara Sauce)
ACTIVE TIME: **55 minutes**

1 teaspoon olive oil
½ cup chopped yellow onion
2 garlic cloves, minced
8 ounces cremini mushrooms (or button mushrooms), diced
One 15-ounce can red beans, rinsed and drained
¼ cup chopped fresh parsley
¾ cup vegan panko bread crumbs (gluten-free if necessary), plus more if needed
2 tablespoons nutritional yeast (or use more bread crumbs)
2 tablespoons liquid aminos (use coconut aminos to be soy-free)
1½ teaspoons dried basil
1½ teaspoons dried oregano
Salt and black pepper to taste
Smoked Gouda Cheese Sauce, Melty Variation (see Tip)
12 ounces spaghetti or other pasta (gluten-free if necessary), optional

4 cups Sun-Dried Tomato Marinara Sauce (or store-bought vegan marinara sauce)

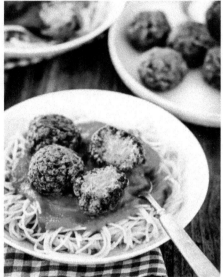

1. Heat the olive oil in a large shallow saucepan over medium heat. Add the onion, garlic, and mushrooms and sauté until the mushrooms are browned and tender and the onions are translucent. Remove from the heat. Transfer to a food processor along with the beans and parsley and pulse until combined and the mixture is mostly uniform, but still a bit chunky.

2. Transfer to a large bowl along with the bread crumbs, nutritional yeast, liquid aminos, basil, oregano, salt, and pepper. Stir with a spoon or use your hands to make sure the mixture is thoroughly combined. It should stick together when squeezed. If it's still too wet, add more bread crumbs.

3. Preheat the oven to 375°F. Line a baking sheet with parchment paper or a silicone baking mat.

4. Scoop up 1 tablespoon of the mixture and roll it into a ball. Use your finger to press a little hole in the middle and shape the mixture into a tiny "bowl." Scoop ½ to ¾ teaspoon of the cheese sauce into the "bowl." Take another tablespoon of the meatball mixture, shape it into a ball, then slightly flatten it into a "dome." Place the dome on top of the meatball bowl, then use your fingers to seal the edges and shape it again into a ball. Place on the baking sheet and repeat with the remaining mixture.

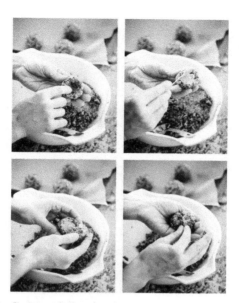

5. Bake for 30 to 35 minutes, flipping once halfway through.

6. While the meatballs are in the oven, cook the pasta (if using): Bring a large pot of water to a boil and add the pasta. Cook according to the package instructions until al dente. Drain and set aside.

7. Heat the marinara sauce while the meatballs are baking.

8. Serve the meatballs on their own, covered in sauce, or on top of the pasta. Leftover meatballs and sauce will keep in an airtight container in the fridge for 3 to 4 days.

TIP

▷ It's best to use the cheese after it's been cooked and allowed to rest for a while (or even chilled). If you have some leftover cheese from the _Avocado Melt_ or French Onion Soup, it would be perfect for this dish since it's already thickened and firmed up a bit. If you don't have any leftover cheese, make it while you're cooking the vegetables (step 1) and let it rest or chill until ready to use.

VARIATION

▷ You can also try using the melty variation of any of the other _Basic Cashew Cheese Sauce_ flavors. They'll each add their own flair to the dish.

Ultimate Twice-Baked Potatoes

SERVES 4

PREP TIME: **10 minutes** (not including time to make Smoked Gouda Cheese Sauce and Quick Bacon Crumbles)
ACTIVE TIME: **20 minutes**
INACTIVE TIME: **70 minutes**

4 large russet potatoes, scrubbed and dried
Olive oil spray
8 ounces cremini mushrooms (or button mushrooms), sliced
2 tablespoons vegan butter (soy-free if necessary)
½ cup unsweetened nondairy milk (soy-free if necessary)
1 teaspoon dried thyme
1 teaspoon dried parsley
1 teaspoon onion powder
1 teaspoon garlic powder
Salt and black pepper to taste
¾ cup chopped green onions (green and white parts)
Smoked Gouda Cheese Sauce (see page
Quick Bacon Crumbles

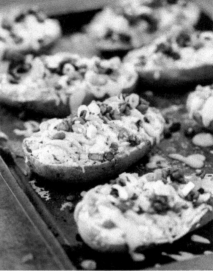

1. Preheat the oven to 400°F. Line a baking sheet with parchment paper or a silicone baking mat. Place the potatoes on the baking sheet and stab a fork into them about four times each to create holes for steam to escape. Spray them with olive oil. Bake for 1 hour, then remove from the oven and let cool. Reduce the heat to 350°F.

2. While the potatoes are baking, heat a large frying pan over medium heat. Brown the mushroom slices, stirring occasionally, for 10 to 12 minutes. When they're done, they should be tender and golden brown. Remove from the heat and set aside.

3. When they're cool enough to handle, slice the potatoes in half lengthwise. Use a spoon to scoop out the insides of each half into a large bowl, leaving a very thin layer close to the skin to help the skin hold its shape. Mash the potatoes until mostly smooth with small chunks. Add the butter, milk, thyme, parsley, onion powder, garlic powder, salt, and pepper and stir until combined. Fold the mushrooms and ½ cup of the green onions into the mixture.

4. Scoop the mixture back into the hollowed-out skins. Return them to the oven and bake for another 20 minutes. Remove from the oven. Drizzle cashew cheese over each potato, then sprinkle the bacon crumbles and the remaining green onions on top. Serve immediately. Keep any leftovers in an airtight container in the fridge for 1 to 2 days.

Double-Double Cheeseburgers

SERVES 4

PREP TIME: **25 minutes** (not including time to make Basic Cashew Cheese Sauce)
ACTIVE TIME: **30 minutes** INACTIVE TIME: **20 minutes**

1 teaspoon olive oil
½ medium yellow onion, chopped
2 garlic cloves, minced
8 ounces cremini mushrooms (or button mushrooms), sliced
2 cups cooked lentils
2 tablespoons liquid aminos (or gluten-free tamari; use coconut aminos to be soy-free)
2 tablespoons nutritional yeast
1 tablespoon vegan Worcestershire sauce (gluten-free and/or soy-free if necessary), optional
1 teaspoon ground cumin
1 teaspoon dried parsley
½ teaspoon smoked paprika
½ teaspoon salt
Black pepper to taste
1 cup rolled oats (certified gluten-free if necessary), plus more if needed
½ cup quinoa flour
3 tablespoons almond flour
2 tablespoons flax meal
4 vegan burger buns (gluten-free if necessary)
 Basic Cashew Cheese Sauce

Optional burger fixings: ketchup, mustard (gluten-free if necessary), vegan mayonnaise (soy-free if necessary), relish, lettuce, sliced tomatoes, sliced red onion, pickles

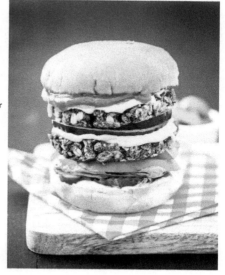

1. Preheat the oven to 375°F. Line a baking sheet with parchment paper or a silicone baking mat.

2. Heat the oil in a large frying pan over medium heat. Add the onion, garlic, and mushrooms and sauté until the mushrooms are tender and the onions are translucent, 4 to 5 minutes. Remove from the heat and transfer to a food processor. Add 1 cup of the lentils, the liquid aminos, nutritional yeast, Worcestershire sauce (if using), cumin, parsley, paprika, salt, and pepper. Pulse until fully combined and all pieces are similar in size.

3. Transfer to a large bowl. Add the remaining lentils, the oats, quinoa flour, almond flour, and flax meal and mix until a thick dough forms. If it's too liquidy, add more oats. If it's too dry, add water by the tablespoon until it's no longer crumbly. It should hold together without crumbling when squeezed.

4. Use your hands to form the mixture into 8 patties and place them on the baking sheet. Bake for 20 minutes, flipping once halfway through to ensure even cooking. Drizzle cheese sauce over the tops and bake for another 5 minutes.

5. To assemble, spread ketchup, mustard, mayonnaise, and/or relish on the top and bottom halves of the buns. Place some lettuce on the bottom bun and stack two patties on top. Top the patties with tomato, red onion, and/or pickles, as desired. Serve immediately. Leftover burgers will keep in an airtight container in the fridge for 4 to 5 days.

57

Beer-Marinated Portobello Tacos with Avocado-Corn Salsa

MAKE 8 TACOS

PREP TIME: **25 minutes**
ACTIVE TIME: **35 minutes**
INACTIVE TIME: **15 minutes**

1½ cups vegan pale or blonde ale (Ground Breaker Brewing IPA No. 5 and Brunehaut Bio Blonde are both vegan and gluten-free)
Juice of 1 lime
1 teaspoon ground cumin
½ teaspoon garlic powder
4 portobello mushrooms, stemmed, gills scraped, cut into 1-inch slices
Sunflower oil, for cooking
6 to 8 corn tortillas (or small flour tortillas)

avocado-corn salsa

2 avocados, pitted, peeled, and diced
1 cup corn kernels (fresh or thawed frozen)
1 cup chopped fresh cilantro
½ cup chopped red onion
2 tablespoons lime juice
1 tablespoon chopped jalapeño
Salt to taste, optional

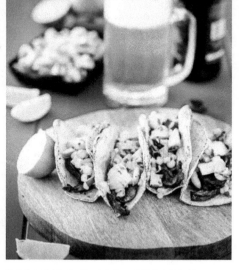

1. Combine the beer, lime juice, cumin, and garlic powder in a shallow baking dish. Add the portobello strips and toss to fully coat. Marinate for 30 minutes, moving the strips around every 10 minutes.

2. While the portobello strips are marinating, **make the salsa:** Combine all the ingredients in a bowl, cover, and chill until ready to use.

3. Heat a large frying pan, preferably cast iron, over medium heat. Add a couple of teaspoons of oil and tilt the pan around to evenly coat the bottom. Add about half of the portobello strips and cook for 10 to 15 minutes, turning every few minutes, until tender and slightly charred, and most of the liquid has been absorbed. Transfer the strips to a plate or bowl and cover with aluminum foil. Add another couple of teaspoons of oil to the pan and repeat with the remaining strips.

4. Heat a griddle or frying pan over medium heat (or just clean the pan you cooked the portobello strips in and reuse it). Cook the tortillas for 30 to 60 seconds on each side, placing them on a plate and covering with aluminum foil when they're done.

5. To serve, place a few portobello strips in a tortilla and top with the avocado-corn salsa. Leftovers will keep in the fridge in separate airtight containers for up to 4 days.

Lazy Vegan Chile Relleno Casserole

SERVES 3 OR 4

PREP TIME: **10 minutes** (not including time to make Basic Cashew or Pepperjack Cheese Sauce)
ACTIVE TIME: **20 minutes**
INACTIVE TIME: **45 minutes**

Olive oil spray
6 canned whole green chiles (from three 4-ounce cans
or the equivalent), rinsed and drained
1 corn tortilla, plus more for serving
One 14-ounce block extra firm tofu, drained
¼ cup unsweetened nondairy milk
1 tablespoon olive oil
⅓ cup unbleached all-purpose flour (or gluten-free flour
blend)
2 tablespoons cornmeal (certified gluten-free if
necessary)
1 teaspoon baking powder
1½ teaspoons ground cumin
1 teaspoon ground coriander
1 teaspoon onion powder
1 teaspoon garlic powder
½ teaspoon salt
¼ teaspoon black pepper

Basic Cashew or Pepperjack Cheese Sauce

Chopped fresh cilantro, optional

Salsa, optional

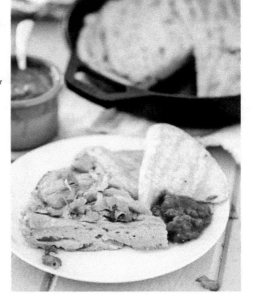

1. Preheat the oven to 375°F . Lightly spray a 10-inch round pan with olive oil.

2. Slice the chiles in half lengthwise and clean the insides of any remaining seeds. Slice the halves in half lengthwise, then slice all of the strips in half crosswise. Set aside.

3. Slice the tortilla in half. then slice each half into about twelve strips. Set aside.

4. Combine the tofu, milk, and olive oil in a food processor and process until smooth.

5. In a large bowl, whisk together the flour, cornmeal, baking powder, cumin, coriander, onion powder, garlic powder, salt, and pepper. Add the pureed tofu and stir until combined. Fold in the chiles and tortilla strips.

6. Spread the mixture in the prepared pan and drizzle cheese sauce over the top (using as much or as little as you'd like). Bake for 35 minutes, or until firm. Remove from the oven and let rest for 10 minutes before serving. Serve topped with cilantro and salsa (if using), and alongside cooked corn tortillas (see the directions under Beer-Marinated Portobello Tacos with Avocado-Corn Salsa). Leftovers will keep in an airtight container in the fridge for 2 to 3 days.

Jackfruit Carnitas Burrito Bowl

SERVES 4

PREP TIME: **30 minutes** (not including time to cook rice and make Pickled Red Cabbage & Onion Relish)
ACTIVE TIME: **45 minutes**
INACTIVE TIME: **60 minutes**

jackfruit carnitas

One 20-ounce can jackfruit (packed in water or brine, not syrup), rinsed and drained
1 tablespoon olive oil
½ medium sweet onion, diced
2 garlic cloves, minced
1 chipotle chile in adobo sauce, chopped
1 teaspoon dried oregano
1 teaspoon ground cumin
1 teaspoon ancho chile powder
½ teaspoon ground coriander
½ teaspoon paprika
1½ cups low-sodium vegetable broth
Juice of 1 lime
2 tablespoons maple syrup
Salt and black pepper to taste

lime crema

½ cup raw cashews, soaked in warm water for at least 1 hour and drained, water reserved
3 tablespoons reserved soaking water
3 tablespoons lime juice
1 tablespoon vegan mayonnaise (soy-free if necessary)
Salt to taste

bowl

3 cups cooked white rice (or brown rice)
One 15-ounce can black beans, rinsed and drained
1 cup chopped fresh cilantro
2 tablespoon lime juice
Salt and black pepper to taste
4 handfuls chopped lettuce (or baby greens)
2 cups halved cherry tomatoes
2 avocados, pitted, peeled, and sliced
Pickled Red Cabbage & Onion Relish

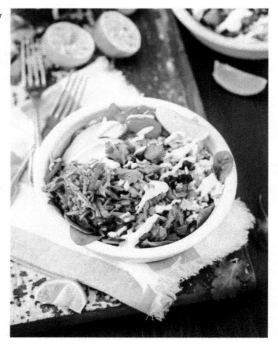

1. Use your fingers or a fork to pull apart the jackfruit until it resembles shredded meat. Don't worry about the seeds—those will soften and break apart as they cook. Set aside.

2. Heat the olive oil in a large shallow saucepan or Dutch oven. Add the onion and garlic and sauté until the onion is translucent. Add the jackfruit and chipotle and cook, stirring occasionally, until the jack-fruit begins to stick to the pan, 5 to 7 minutes.

3. Add the oregano, cumin, ancho chile powder, coriander, and paprika and stir until combined. Cook for about 2 minutes. Add the broth, lime juice, and maple syrup. Bring to a boil, then reduce to a simmer. Cover and cook for about 15 minutes, stirring a few times, until the liquid has been absorbed and the jackfruit is starting to stick to the pan. Remove from the heat and add salt and pepper.

4. While the jackfruit is cooking, **make the lime crema** : Combine the crema ingredients in a food processor and process until smooth, pausing to scrape the sides as needed. Chill until ready to use.

5. Combine the rice and beans in a pot (if you just cooked the rice, simply add the beans to the rice in the pot) and cook over medium heat for a few minutes, until heated through. Remove from the heat and add the cilantro, lime juice, salt and pepper.

6. To serve, fill four bowls with a handful of lettuce each. Add cilantro rice and beans, jackfruit carnitas, cherry tomatoes, and avocado to each bowl. Drizzle each with lime crema, then garnish with a generous pile of relish. Serve immediately.

VARIATION

▷ If you prefer burritos (who can blame you?), feel free to stuff a tortilla with all these ingredients.

BALANCED VEGAN

VEGAN MEALS THAT HEALTH NUTS CAN GET EXCITED ABOUT

Chinese Chickpea Salad

SERVES 4 TO 6

PREP TIME: **20 minutes**
ACTIVE TIME: **15 minutes**

1 tablespoon sesame oil
3 cups cooked chickpeas (or two 15-ounce cans, rinsed and drained)
3 tablespoons gluten-free tamari (use coconut aminos to be soy-free)
4 cups shredded napa cabbage (about 1 small head)
1 cup shredded red cabbage
1 cup grated carrots (3 or 4 large carrots)
1 cup toasted sliced almonds
½ cup sliced green onions (green and white parts)
One 10-ounce can mandarin oranges (preferably packed in juice, not syrup), rinsed and drained
One 8-ounce can sliced water chestnuts, rinsed, drained, and cut in half
Crispy rice crackers, crumbled

miso ginger dressing
½ cup rice vinegar
2 tablespoons sesame oil
2 tablespoons maple syrup
1 tablespoon white soy miso (or chickpea miso)
2 teaspoons freshly grated ginger

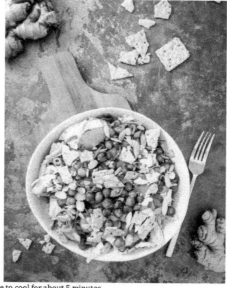

1. Heat the sesame oil in a large shallow saucepan over medium heat. Add the chickpeas and cook for a couple of minutes. Add the tamari and cook, stirring occasionally, until the liquid has been absorbed. Set aside to cool for about 5 minutes.

2. **To make the dressing** : Stir together all the ingredients in a cup or small bowl.

3. Combine the napa cabbage, red cabbage, carrots, almonds, green onions, mandarin oranges, and water chestnuts in a large bowl. Add the chickpeas and dressing and toss until fully combined. Serve immediately, topped with crumbled rice crackers.

TIP

▶ You can prep this ahead of time by preparing the chickpeas, the salad (without the almonds), and the dressing and storing them separately. Combine the three elements, plus the almonds, just before serving.

Pecan Pesto Spaghetti Squash with Peas & Kale

SERVES 4 TO 6

PREP TIME: **15 minutes** (not including time to make Pepita Parmesan)
ACTIVE TIME: **20 minutes**
INACTIVE TIME: **35 minutes**

1 medium (2-pound) spaghetti squash, halved lengthwise, seeds removed
Olive oil spray
Salt and black pepper to taste
1 teaspoon olive oil
1 shallot, chopped
1 bunch (12 to 16 ounces) kale, stems removed, chopped
1½ cups green peas (fresh or thawed frozen)
 Pepita Parmesan, optional

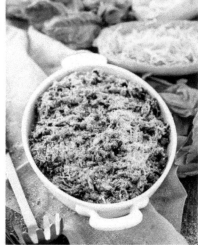

pecan pesto
½ cup pecan pieces
2 garlic cloves
2 cups loosely packed chopped greens of your choice (spinach, kale, or chard)
1 cup loosely packed chopped fresh basil
3 tablespoons low-sodium vegetable broth (or water)
3 tablespoons olive oil
2 tablespoons lemon juice
Salt and black pepper to taste

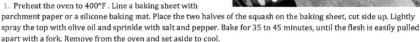

1. Preheat the oven to 400°F . Line a baking sheet with parchment paper or a silicone baking mat. Place the two halves of the squash on the baking sheet, cut side up. Lightly spray the top with olive oil and sprinkle with salt and pepper. Bake for 35 to 45 minutes, until the flesh is easily pulled apart with a fork. Remove from the oven and set aside to cool.

2. While the squash is roasting, **make the pesto** : Combine all the ingredients in a food processor and process until mostly smooth (teeny chunks or pieces are okay), pausing to scrape the sides as needed. Set aside until ready to use.

3. Once the squash is cool enough to touch, use a fork to tear the flesh into spaghetti-like strands.

4. Heat the olive oil in a large shallow saucepan over medium heat. Add the shallot and cook until just translucent. Add the kale, peas, and squash strands and cook, stirring occasionally, until the kale begins to wilt. Stir in the pesto sauce. Taste and add salt and pepper if necessary. Serve immediately, topped with Pepita Parmesan, if desired. Keep leftovers in an airtight container in the fridge for up to 2 days.

VARIATIONS

▶ In the mood for pasta? Replace the spaghetti squash with cooked pasta of your choice. Rice would be another good option. In either case, pick up the recipe at step 2, making the pesto.

▶ To make this oil-free, you can replace all the olive oil with low-sodium vegetable broth or water.

Chile-Roasted Tofu Lettuce Cups

SERVES 4

PREP TIME: **15 minutes** (not including time to make Lemon Tahini Sauce)
ACTIVE TIME: **20 minutes**
INACTIVE TIME: **45 minutes**

chile-roasted tofu

One 14-ounce block extra firm tofu, pressed for at least
1 hour (see _How to Press Tofu_)
¼ cup orange juice
1 tablespoon coconut oil, melted
1 tablespoon ancho chile powder
2 teaspoons maple syrup
½ teaspoon garlic powder
2 pinches of cayenne pepper
½ teaspoon salt

lettuce cups

1 large or 2 small heads butter lettuce, separated into
individual leaves (see Tip)
Lemon Tahini Sauce

1 large carrot, peeled and grated
½ red bell pepper, sliced into long, thin slivers
15 to 20 chives, trimmed
White or black sesame seeds

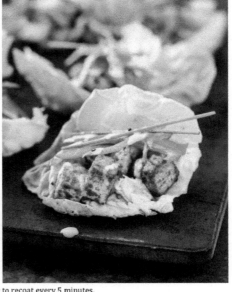

1. **To make the tofu** : Slice the tofu horizontally so
that you have two flat sheets. Dice both sheets into ½-
inch cubes.

2. In a shallow baking dish, combine the orange juice,
coconut oil, ancho chile powder, maple syrup, garlic
powder, cayenne pepper, and salt. Add the tofu cubes
and toss to coat. Marinate for about 20 minutes, tossing to recoat every 5 minutes.

3. Preheat the oven to 400°F . Line a baking sheet with parchment paper or a silicone baking mat. Spread out the tofu
on the baking sheet. Bake for 25 minutes, or until the edges are crispy and browned, flipping once halfway through to
ensure even cooking. Remove from the oven.

4. To serve, fill a lettuce leaf with a large spoonful of the tofu. Drizzle with tahini sauce. Top with a pinch of carrot, a
couple of slivers of red bell pepper, and 1 to 2 chives. Sprinkle with sesame seeds. Leftover tofu will keep in an airtight
container in the fridge for 3 to 4 days.

TIP

▶ To prevent the lettuce leaves from tearing or falling apart when you're removing them from the head, slice the base off the head first.

Buddha Bowl

SERVES 4

PREP TIME: **10 minutes** (not including time to make Pickled Red Cabbage & Onion Relish and Lemon Tahini Sauce or Avocado Ranch Dressing)
ACTIVE TIME: **40 minutes**

2 medium sweet potatoes or yams, peeled and chopped into 1-inch cubes
Olive oil spray
2 pinches of smoked paprika
Salt and black pepper to taste
3 cups water
1½ cups roasted buckwheat groats (kasha)
2 to 3 cups chopped spinach
1½ cups cooked, warm kidney beans (or one 15-ounce) can, rinsed and drained; or use another bean of your choice)
1 cucumber, sliced
1 avocado, pitted, peeled, and sliced
 Pickled Red Cabbage & Onion Relish

Lemon Tahini Sauce or Avocado Ranch Dressing

⅓ cup toasted pepitas (pumpkin seeds)

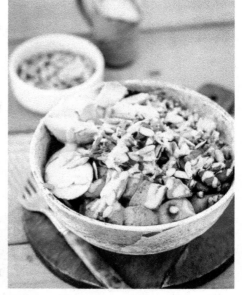

1. Preheat the oven to 425°F. Line a baking sheet with parchment paper or a silicone baking mat. Spread out the sweet potato cubes on the pan and spray with olive oil. Add the paprika, salt, and pepper and toss to coat. Bake for 30 minutes, or until tender and browned, tossing once halfway through to ensure even cooking. Set aside to cool.

2. While the sweet potatoes are cooking, cook the buckwheat groats: Bring the water to a boil in a medium pot. Add the buckwheat groats and return to a boil. Reduce the heat, cover, and simmer until most of the water has been absorbed, 11 to 12 minutes. Remove from the heat and add salt.

3. To serve, fill each bowl with spinach, buckwheat groats, beans, sweet potato, cucumber, avocado, and cabbage relish. Drizzle with dressing and top with toasted pepitas.

VARIATION

▶ You can switch out the buckwheat groats with 3 cups cooked grain of your choice, such as rice, quinoa, millet, amaranth, or even farro (though that won't be gluten-free).

Beet Hummus Collard Wraps

SERVES 4 TO 6

PREP TIME: **15 minutes**
ACTIVE TIME: **20 minutes**
INACTIVE TIME: **20 minutes**

beet hummus

1 large beet, peeled and chopped
1½ cups cooked chickpeas (or one 15-ounce can, rinsed and drained)
2 tablespoons tahini (gluten-free if necessary)
2 tablespoons olive oil
2 tablespoons lemon juice
1 garlic clove, peeled
Pinch of smoked paprika
Salt and black pepper to taste

wraps

6 large collard leaves, cleaned, dried, stems removed
2 carrots, peeled and julienned
1 yellow bell pepper, sliced
1 avocado, pitted, peeled, and sliced
Bean sprouts (or other sprouts)

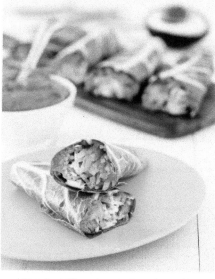

1. Place the beet in a small pot and cover with water. Bring to a boil, then reduce to a simmer and cover. Cook until the beet is tender enough to be easily pierced by a fork, 8 to 10 minutes. Remove from the heat.

2. Use a slotted spoon to transfer the beet to a food processor (reserving the cooking water) and add the chickpeas, tahini, olive oil, lemon juice, garlic, and paprika. Process until smooth, pausing to scrape the sides as necessary. If it's too thick, add beet water by the tablespoon until it reaches your desired consistency. Taste and add salt and pepper as needed. Chill for 30 minutes or until ready to use.

3. Lay a collard leaf flat, bottom up, and carefully run a knife down the spine of the stem, shaving off the bulk of the thick stem. Spread some beet hummus on the leaf, leaving about an inch around the perimeter. On one half of the leaf, parallel to the spine, lay out a small bit of carrots, bell pepper, and avocado slices, then top with a small pile of sprouts. Starting with that edge (the one nearest the fillings), roll the collard leaf over the filling and continue to roll, tucking in the filling as needed, until the leaf is completely rolled up. Slice in half and place on a plate, seam side down. Repeat with the remaining leaves. Serve immediately. Leftover hummus will keep in an airtight container in the fridge for 4 to 5 days.

Green Quinoa Salad

PREP TIME: **25 minutes** (not including time to cook quinoa)
ACTIVE TIME: **20 minutes**

1 pound brussels sprouts
½ cup diced yellow onion
1 garlic clove, minced
1 tablespoon water, plus more if necessary
1½ cups diced zucchini
1½ cups shelled edamame
¼ cup lemon juice
1 tablespoon grated lemon zest
1 tablespoon maple syrup
3 cups cooked quinoa
3 cups chopped chard leaves
½ cup chopped fresh basil
½ cup chopped pistachios
Salt and black pepper to taste

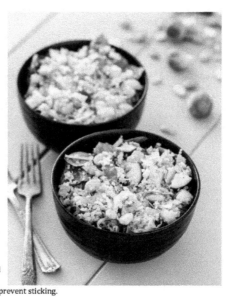

1. Slice a brussels sprout in half lengthwise through the stem. Turn each half cut side down and thinly slice into shreds. Repeat with all of the brussels sprouts. Set aside.

2. Heat a large shallow saucepan over medium heat. Add the onion, garlic, and water and cook until the onion is just becoming translucent. Add more water as needed to prevent sticking.

3. Add the brussels sprouts, zucchini, and edamame. Cook for about 3 minutes, until the brussels sprouts are just beginning to wilt. Remove from the heat and stir in the lemon juice, lemon zest, and maple syrup.

4. Stir in the quinoa, chard, basil, and pistachios. Taste and add salt and pepper if needed. Serve immediately or chill until ready to serve. Leftovers will keep in an airtight container in the fridge for 3 to 4 days.

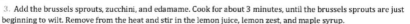

No-Bake Zucchini Manicotti

SERVES 3 OR 4

PREP TIME: **15 minutes** (not including time to make Sun-Dried Tomato Marinara Sauce and Pepita Parmesan)
ACTIVE TIME: **15 minutes**
INACTIVE TIME: **60 minutes**

2 large zucchini
Salt
Sun-Dried Tomato Marinara ; or store-bought vegan marinara sauce
Pepita Parmesan , optional
½ cup loosely packed basil chiffonade

herbed macadamia ricotta

1 cup raw macadamia nuts, soaked in warm water for at least 1 hour and drained, water reserved
3 tablespoons reserved soaking water
2 tablespoons lemon juice
1 teaspoon dried basil
1 teaspoon dried oregano
¾ teaspoon salt
½ teaspoon white soy miso (or chickpea miso)

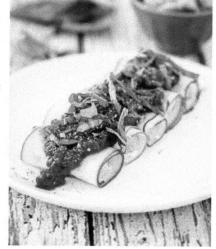

1. Trim the ends of the zucchini. Use a vegetable peeler or mandoline to slice down the length of the zucchini, making long, thin strips. Lay out the zucchini strips on a couple of paper towels. Sprinkle with salt and let drain for about 10 minutes. The salt will help the zucchini release excess water and soften.

2. While the zucchini is draining, **make the herbed ricotta** : Combine the macadamia nuts, 4 teaspoons of the reserved soaking water, the lemon juice, dried basil, oregano, salt, and miso in a food processor and process until smooth, pausing to scrape the sides as needed. If you have a hard time getting the cheese to move, you may need to add more of the soaking water a teaspoon at a time until it moves more smoothly.

3. Pat the zucchini dry with a clean kitchen towel. Lay out two slices of zucchini, one overlapping the other by about half. Scoop 1 scant tablespoon ricotta onto one end of the strips. Take the ends of the zucchini closest to the ricotta and carefully roll them over the ricotta. Continue until completely rolled up. Place on a plate seam side down. Repeat with the remaining zucchini slices.

4. Heat the marinara sauce. Serve the manicotti topped with sauce, Pepita Parmesan (if using), and basil chiffonade. Keep any leftover ricotta in an airtight container in the fridge for up to 7 days.

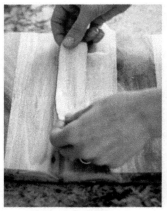
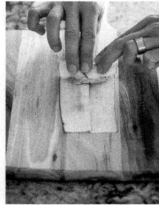
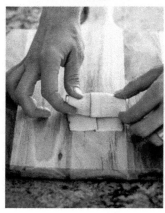

HOMESTYLE VEGAN

HOMESTYLE VEGAN FOOD "JUST LIKE MOM MAKES IT"

Chickpea & Dumplin' Soup

SERVES 6 TO 8

PREP TIME: **15 minutes**
ACTIVE TIME: **40 minutes** INACTIVE TIME: **15 minutes**

5 tablespoons cold vegan butter (soy-free if necessary)
1 small yellow onion, diced
4 celery stalks, sliced
3 large carrots, peeled and sliced
2 garlic cloves, minced
8 ounces cremini mushrooms (or button mushrooms), sliced
3 bay leaves
2½ teaspoons dried thyme
2 teaspoons dried rosemary
1 teaspoon dried parsley
½ teaspoon ground cumin
¼ cup oat flour (or other flour; certified gluten-free if necessary)
3 cups cooked chickpeas or two 15-ounce cans, rinsed and drained
1 quart vegetable broth
1¼ cups unbleached all-purpose flour (or gluten-free flour blend, soy-free if necessary)
½ cup fine cornmeal (certified gluten-free if necessary)
2 teaspoons baking powder
1 teaspoon baking soda
Salt and black pepper to taste
¼ teaspoon garlic powder
¼ teaspoon xanthan gum (exclude if using all-purpose flour or if your gluten-free blend includes it)
¾ cup unsweetened nondairy milk (nut-free and/or soy-free if necessary)
2 tablespoons chopped fresh parsley

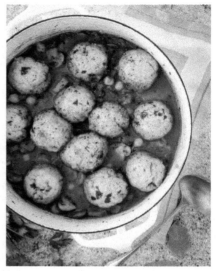

1. Melt 1 tablespoon of the butter over medium heat in a large Dutch oven or pot (choose a wide one to give you more dumpling surface area). Add the onion, celery, carrot, and garlic and cook for about 3 minutes. Add the mushrooms and cook for 3 minutes more, stirring occasionally. Stir in the bay leaves, 2 teaspoons of the thyme, the rosemary, dried parsley, and cumin and cook for 1 minute. Add the oat flour and stir until the flour is no longer visible. Add the chickpeas and broth, bring to a boil, then reduce to a simmer. Cover and cook for about 10 minutes, stirring every few minutes to prevent sticking.

2. In a large bowl, combine the all-purpose flour, cornmeal, baking powder, baking soda, ½ teaspoon salt, the garlic powder, and xanthan gum (if using). Add the remaining butter and use a pastry cutter or a fork to cut the butter into the flour mixture until you have a coarse meal, similar to the texture of wet sand. In a cup or small bowl, combine the milk and fresh parsley. Pour over the flour mixture. Stir until you have a thick dough.

3. Uncover the pot and remove the bay leaves. Add salt and pepper. Drop the dough into the soup in 8 to 10 large spoonfuls. Space the dumplings evenly, keeping in mind that they'll expand. Cover and cook for 15 minutes more, or until the dumplings are solid. Sprinkle with more pepper. Serve immediately. Leftovers will keep in an airtight container in the fridge for 2 to 3 days.

Shiitake Stroganoff

SERVES 4

PREP TIME: **30 minutes**
ACTIVE TIME: **25 minutes**

12 ounces spiral pasta (gluten-free if necessary)
One 12-ounce vacuum-packed block extra firm silken tofu
3 tablespoons lemon juice
1 tablespoon unsweetened nondairy milk (nut-free if necessary)
2 teaspoons white wine vinegar
1 teaspoon olive oil
4 shallots, chopped
1 garlic clove, minced
1 pound shiitake mushrooms, stemmed and sliced (see Variation)
½ cup vegan white wine (or low-sodium vegetable broth)
2 teaspoons nutritional yeast, optional
1 teaspoon paprika
1 cup chopped fresh parsley
Salt and black pepper to taste

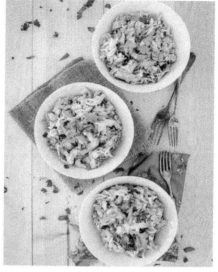

1. Bring a large pot of water to a boil and add the pasta. Cook according to the package instructions until al dente. Drain and set aside.

2. Combine the tofu, lemon juice, milk, and vinegar in a food processor and process until smooth. Set aside.

3. Heat the olive oil in a large shallow saucepan over medium heat. Add the shallots and garlic and sauté until the shallots are almost translucent.

4. Add the mushrooms and cook, stirring occasionally, until the mushrooms are tender, 10 to 12 minutes. Add the wine and cook until the liquid has been absorbed. Stir in the nutritional yeast and paprika.

5. Add the reserved tofu mixture and cook until heated through. Add the parsley, salt, and pepper. Fold in the pasta and serve immediately. Refrigerate any leftovers in an airtight container for up to 3 days.

VARIATION

▶ You can use other types of mushrooms, or even a mixture of mushrooms, to replace the shiitakes.

Unstuffed Cabbage Rolls

SERVES 8

PREP TIME: **30 minutes** (not including time to cook brown rice)
ACTIVE TIME: **20 minutes**
INACTIVE TIME: **30 minutes**

Olive oil spray
1 large (2- to 3-pound) head cabbage, quartered and cored
1 teaspoon olive oil
1 medium sweet onion, diced
2 garlic cloves, minced
1 red bell pepper, diced
3 cups cooked black beans or two 15-ounce cans, rinsed and drained
One 15-ounce can no-salt-added fire-roasted diced tomatoes
2 tablespoons no-salt-added tomato paste
2 tablespoons liquid aminos (or gluten-free tamari; use coconut aminos to be soy-free)
1 teaspoon dried parsley
1 teaspoon dried oregano
½ teaspoon ground cumin
½ teaspoon paprika
1½ cups cooked brown rice (or other grain)
2 tablespoons nutritional yeast
2 tablespoons lemon juice
Salt and black pepper to taste

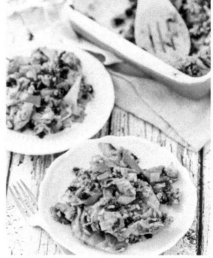

1. Preheat the oven to 375°F. Lightly spray a 9 × 13-inch baking dish with olive oil.

2. Chop each cabbage quarter into 1-inch strips. Set aside.

3. Heat the olive oil in a large shallow saucepan over medium heat. Add the onion and garlic and sauté until the onion is just becoming translucent.

4. Add the bell pepper, black beans, tomatoes with their juice, tomato paste, liquid aminos, parsley, oregano, cumin, and paprika. Cover and cook, stirring occasionally, until the bell pepper is tender.

5. Add the cabbage, cover again, and cook until the cabbage is soft. Stir in the rice and cook until heated through. Add the nutritional yeast, lemon juice, salt, and pepper. Remove from the heat.

6. Transfer to the baking dish and bake, uncovered, for 25 minutes. Let cool for a few minutes before serving. Leftovers will keep in an airtight container in the fridge for 4 to 5 days.

Not-Tuna Casserole

SERVES 6 TO 8

PREP TIME: **5 minutes** (not including time to make Cream of Mushroom Soup)
ACTIVE TIME: **20 minutes**
INACTIVE TIME: **20 minutes**

Olive oil spray
1 pound pasta (gluten-free if necessary)
1 teaspoon olive oil
½ yellow onion, diced
1½ cups cooked chickpeas (or one 15-ounce can, rinsed and drained)
One 14- to 15-ounce can artichoke hearts, rinsed, drained, and quartered if whole
1 teaspoon dried thyme
½ teaspoon garlic powder
Salt and black pepper to taste
Cream of Mushroom Soup

2 cups lightly crushed plain kettle-style potato chips, optional

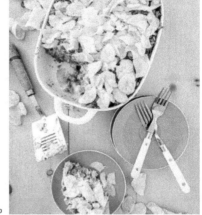

1. Preheat the oven to 350°F. Lightly spray a 9 × 13-inch baking dish with olive oil.

2. Bring a pot of water to a boil and cook the pasta according to the package instructions until al dente. Drain and rinse with cold water.

3. While the pasta is cooking, heat the olive oil in a large shallow saucepan over medium heat. Add the onion and sauté until translucent. Add the chickpeas and artichokes and cook for about 5 minutes, using your spatula to tear apart the artichokes as they cook. Add the thyme and garlic powder.

4. Use a potato masher to gently mash the chickpeas and artichokes until just slightly mashed with chunks. Add the soup and pasta and stir until combined. Add salt and pepper.

5. Remove from the heat, transfer to the prepared baking dish, and bake for 15 minutes. Sprinkle the potato chips over the top (if using) and bake for another 5 minutes. Serve immediately. Leftovers will keep in an airtight container in the fridge for 2 to 3 days.

BBQ-Glazed Tempeh

SERVES 4

PREP TIME: **3 minutes**
ACTIVE TIME: **20 minutes**

One 8-ounce package tempeh
1 tablespoon olive oil
⅔ cup vegan barbecue sauce (homemade or store-bought)
Salt and black pepper to taste

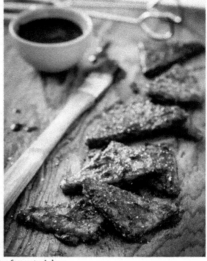

1. Slice the block of tempeh in half horizontally, then slice each half diagonally so that you have four triangles. Slice each of those in half horizontally to get eight triangles (they should all be the same size of the original four triangles).

2. Heat the oil in a large frying pan, preferably cast iron, over medium heat. Add the tempeh triangles and cook for 2 to 3 minutes per side, or until each side has golden cooking marks.

3. Pour half of the sauce over the triangles, spread it to cover them, then flip them over so that they cook in the sauce. Once that sauce has been absorbed, repeat with the remaining sauce. Once all the sauce has been absorbed, remove from the heat and add salt and pepper. Serve immediately. Keep leftovers in an airtight container in the fridge for up to 4 days.

Smoky Shroom Sausage & Red Potato Goulash

SERVES 4 TO 6

PREP TIME: **15 minutes**
ACTIVE TIME: **30 minutes**

2 teaspoons olive oil
1 teaspoon fennel seeds
½ teaspoon ground sage
8 ounces cremini mushrooms, sliced
1 tablespoon liquid aminos (use coconut aminos to be soy-free)
1 teaspoon dried thyme
½ teaspoon dried oregano
½ teaspoon liquid smoke
Salt and black pepper to taste
1 tablespoon vegan butter (soy-free if necessary)
1 small red onion, thinly sliced
2 garlic cloves, minced
1 tablespoon Hungarian paprika (or regular paprika)
3 pounds red potatoes, chopped into 1-inch cubes
1½ cups low-sodium vegetable broth
½ cup chopped fresh parsley
Vegan sour cream (soy-free if necessary), optional

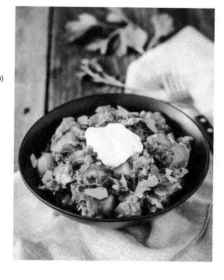

1. Preheat the oven to 200°F.

2. Heat the olive oil in a large shallow saucepan or Dutch oven over medium heat. Add the fennel seeds and sage and cook until fragrant, 2 to 3 minutes.

3. Add the mushrooms and cook for about 1 minute. Add the liquid aminos, thyme, and oregano. Cook until the mushrooms are tender and browned and the liquid has cooked away, about 7 minutes.

4. Add the liquid smoke, salt, and pepper. Spread out the mushrooms on the prepared baking sheet. Roast for 30 minutes or until needed in step 7, whichever is less.

5. While the mushrooms are roasting, melt the butter in the same pan you used to cook the mushrooms. Add the onion and sauté until translucent. Add the garlic and cook for 1 to 2 minutes more, until the garlic is fragrant. Stir in the paprika and cook for 1 minute.

6. Add the potatoes and broth. Bring to a boil, then reduce to a simmer and cover. Cook, stirring occasionally, until tender, 15 to 20 minutes.

7. Add the mushrooms to the potatoes, along with the parsley. Season with more salt and/or pepper if necessary. Serve immediately, topped with vegan sour cream (if using). Leftovers will keep in an airtight container in the fridge for 3 to 4 days.

VEGAN CLASSICS

IMPRESSIVE MEALS THAT WILL LEAVE THEM WITH ONLY GOOD THINGS TO SAY ABOUT YOU

Balsamic-Roasted Beet & Cheese Galette

SERVES 4

PREP TIME: **20 minutes** (not including time to make Mixed Herb Cheese Sauce)
ACTIVE TIME: **70 minutes**
INACTIVE TIME: **40 minutes**

crust

¼ cup unsweetened nondairy milk (soy-free if necessary)
3 tablespoons 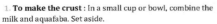 aquafaba
1½ cups unbleached all-purpose flour (or gluten-free flour
blend, soy-free if necessary), plus more for the work surface
1 tablespoon coconut sugar
½ teaspoon salt
½ teaspoon baking soda
½ teaspoon xanthan gum (exclude if using all-purpose flour or
if your gluten-free blend includes it)

8 tablespoons very cold vegan butter (soy-free if
necessary; see Tip)

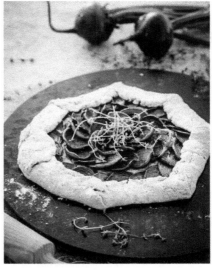

filling

Olive oil spray
2 medium red beets, peeled and very thinly sliced (see Tip)
2 medium golden beets, peeled and very thinly sliced (see Tip)
6 tablespoons balsamic vinegar
2 tablespoons coconut sugar
Salt and black pepper to taste
Mixed Herb Cheese Sauce, 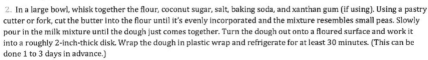 Spread Variation

Fresh thyme leaves

1. **To make the crust** : In a small cup or bowl, combine the milk and aquafaba. Set aside.

2. In a large bowl, whisk together the flour, coconut sugar, salt, baking soda, and xanthan gum (if using). Using a pastry cutter or fork, cut the butter into the flour until it's evenly incorporated and the mixture resembles small peas. Slowly pour in the milk mixture until the dough just comes together. Turn the dough out onto a floured surface and work it into a roughly 2-inch-thick disk. Wrap the dough in plastic wrap and refrigerate for at least 30 minutes. (This can be done 1 to 3 days in advance.)

3. While the dough is chilling, **make the filling** : Preheat the oven to 400°F . Lightly spray two 9 × 13-inch (23 × 33-cm) baking dishes with olive oil. Spread out the red beet slices in one dish and the golden beets in the other (you can do them all in one, but the red beets will stain the golden beets). Drizzle 3 tablespoons of the vinegar over each set of beets, then add 1 tablespoon coconut sugar per dish and top with salt and pepper. Toss to coat, then spread out the slices again (it's okay if they overlap). Bake for about 15 minutes, flipping once halfway through. The beets will be undercooked, which is okay. Remove them from the oven and set aside.

4. Reduce the temperature to 350°F. Line a baking sheet, pizza pan, or pizza stone with parchment paper or a silicone baking mat.

5. Once the dough has chilled for at least 30 minutes, remove it from the refrigerator. Remove the plastic wrap (set it aside for now) and place the dough on a floured surface. Turn it over so both sides are lightly floured. If the dough is

79

hard, knead it lightly with your hands to make it pliable. If it's too dry and begins to crack, sprinkle with a couple of drops of water. Lay the plastic wrap on top of the dough and use a rolling pin to roll it out until it's a circle about 10 inches in diameter and ¼ inch (6 mm) thick. Gently transfer the dough to the prepared baking sheet, pan, or stone. (I do this by scooting a thin, rimless baking sheet under the dough to transport it to the other baking sheet; a pizza peel may also work.)

6. Spread the cheese on top of the dough, leaving about 1½ inches around the perimeter. Lay the beet slices on top of the cheese. You can lay them out willy-nilly or in a pretty pattern—your choice. If there is any liquid in the baking dish, pour it over the beets. Fold the edges of the dough over the beets.

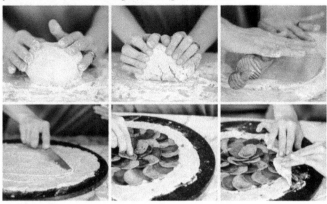

7. Bake for 35 to 40 minutes, until the dough is golden brown. Remove from the oven, slice, and serve topped with fresh thyme. Leftovers will keep in an airtight container in the fridge for up to 2 days.

TIP

▷ About 10 minutes before using vegan butter, stick it in the freezer so it gets extra cold.

▷ When slicing your beets, it's best to use a mandoline to get superthin slices.

80

French Onion Soup

SERVES 6

PREP TIME: **30 minutes** (not including time to make Smoky Gouda Cheese Sauce)
ACTIVE TIME: **60 minutes**

4 tablespoons vegan butter (soy-free if necessary)
6 medium yellow onions, halved and very thinly sliced
2 garlic cloves, minced
1 tablespoon fresh thyme leaves
2 bay leaves
1 cup vegan dry white wine
2 tablespoons oat flour (certified gluten-free if necessary)
2 quarts low-sodium vegetable broth
1 tablespoon nutritional yeast, optional
Salt and black pepper to taste
1 vegan baguette, sliced (gluten-free if necessary)
Smoked Gouda Cheese Sauce, "Melty" Variation (see Tip)
Chopped fresh parsley, optional

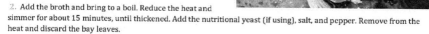
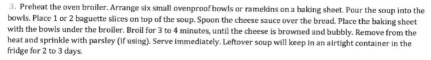

1. Melt the butter in a large pot or Dutch oven over medium heat. Add the onions and cook for 20 to 25 minutes, stirring every so often, until browned and caramelized. Add the garlic, thyme, and bay leaves and cook for 2 to 3 minutes more, until the garlic is fragrant. Add the wine and cook, stirring occasionally, until the liquid has been absorbed. Add the oat flour and cook, stirring constantly, until the flour is no longer visible, about 2 minutes.

2. Add the broth and bring to a boil. Reduce the heat and simmer for about 15 minutes, until thickened. Add the nutritional yeast (if using), salt, and pepper. Remove from the heat and discard the bay leaves.

3. Preheat the oven broiler. Arrange six small ovenproof bowls or ramekins on a baking sheet. Pour the soup into the bowls. Place 1 or 2 baguette slices on top of the soup. Spoon the cheese sauce over the bread. Place the baking sheet with the bowls under the broiler. Broil for 3 to 4 minutes, until the cheese is browned and bubbly. Remove from the heat and sprinkle with parsley (if using). Serve immediately. Leftover soup will keep in an airtight container in the fridge for 2 to 3 days.

TIP

 Heating the cheese sauce will take 5 to 7 minutes, so I suggest preparing it while the soup is simmering.

Truffled Mashed Potato–Stuffed Portobellos

SERVES 4

PREP TIME: **25 minutes** (not including time to cook mashed potatoes)
ACTIVE TIME: **30 minutes**
INACTIVE TIME: **20 minutes**

4 large portobello mushrooms
2 teaspoons vegan butter (soy-free if necessary)
2 shallots, diced
1 garlic clove, minced
2 teaspoons fresh thyme leaves, plus more for garnish
Olive oil spray
Salt and black pepper to taste
½ batch Truffled Mashed Potatoes (see Tip)

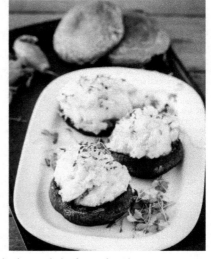

1. Preheat the oven to 375°F . Line a baking sheet with parchment paper or a silicone baking mat.

2. Remove the stems from the portobellos and set aside the caps. Dice the stems into ½-inch pieces. Melt the butter in a large frying pan, preferably cast iron, over medium heat. Add the shallots, garlic, mushroom stems, and thyme. Cook for about 5 minutes, stirring occasionally, until the mushrooms are tender. Remove from the heat.

3. Spray the tops of the portobello caps with olive oil and place gill side up on the baking sheet. Sprinkle with salt and pepper, then divide the stem mixture among them. Scoop heaping mounds of mashed potatoes on top. Bake for 20 minutes, or until the mashed potatoes are golden. Serve immediately, garnished with more thyme leaves.

VARIATION

▶ To fancy up this dish, mash the potatoes until they're very smooth and transfer them to a pastry bag. Pipe the mashed potatoes into the mushroom caps as if you were icing a cupcake. Proceed with the instructions from there.

TIP

▶ If you don't already have the mashed potatoes on hand, prepare them while you preheat the oven.

82

Butternut Squash Risotto with Sage Butter

SERVES 6

PREP TIME: **15 minutes** (not including time to make Pepita Parmesan)
ACTIVE TIME: **50 minutes**

1 butternut squash, peeled, seeded, and chopped into 1-inch cubes
Olive oil spray
2 tablespoons coconut sugar
1 teaspoon ground cinnamon
1 teaspoon ground cumin
Salt and black pepper to taste
6 cups low-sodium vegetable broth
8 tablespoons vegan butter (soy-free if necessary)
1 cup loosely packed fresh sage leaves
4 shallots, diced
1½ cups arborio rice (certified gluten-free if necessary)
½ cup vegan white wine
⅓ cup nutritional yeast
 Pepita Parmesan , optional
Toasted pine nuts, optional

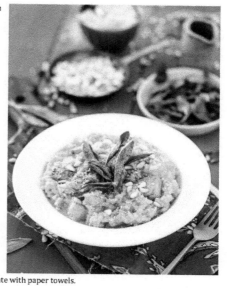

1. Preheat the oven to 425°F. Line a baking sheet with parchment paper or a silicone baking mat. Spread out the squash cubes on the sheet and lightly spray with olive oil. Sprinkle with the coconut sugar, cinnamon, cumin, salt, and pepper. Toss to evenly coat, then spread out again on the sheet. Bake for 25 minutes, or until tender and caramelized. When done, remove from the oven and set aside.

2. Once the squash is in the oven, pour the broth into a pot, bring to a boil, then reduce to a low simmer. Line a plate with paper towels.

3. Melt the butter in a large shallow saucepan or Dutch oven over medium heat. Add the sage leaves and cook for 3 to 5 minutes, stirring occasionally, until the leaves are crispy. Use a slotted spoon to transfer the leaves to the plate. Pour half of the butter into a small cup and set aside.

4. Add the shallots to the butter in the pan and sauté until translucent. Add the rice and cook for a couple of minutes, just until the rice begins to become translucent. Add the wine and cook until the wine is absorbed. Add 2 cups of the broth, cover, and cook until the broth is absorbed. Add another 1 cup broth, cover, and cook until the broth is absorbed. Repeat until all the broth has been used and the rice is tender.

5. Add the nutritional yeast, salt, and pepper. Stir in the squash and remove from the heat. Serve topped with a drizzle of the reserved sage butter, the crispy sage leaves, Pepita Parmesan (if using), and toasted pine nuts (if using). Leftovers will keep in an airtight container in the fridge for 3 to 4 days.

83

Kung Pao Cauliflower

SERVES 4 TO 6

PREP TIME: **20 minutes** (not including time to cook noodles or rice)
ACTIVE TIME: **25 minutes**

kung pao sauce

¼ cup water
2 tablespoons gluten-free tamari (use coconut aminos to be soy-free)
2 tablespoons brown rice vinegar
1 tablespoon no-salt-added tomato paste
2 teaspoons maple syrup
1 teaspoon sriracha, optional
1 teaspoon grated fresh ginger
2 teaspoons arrowroot powder
1 tablespoon sesame oil
1 tablespoon red pepper flakes
1 cup diced sweet onion
1 large (1½- to 2-pound) head cauliflower, broken into small florets
2 tablespoons liquid aminos (or gluten-free tamari; use coconut aminos to be soy-free)
2 garlic cloves, minced
1 red bell pepper, diced
½ cup cashews
5 green onions (white parts chopped, green parts sliced lengthwise into thin strands)
Salt and black pepper to taste, optional
Cooked noodles (gluten-free if necessary) or rice

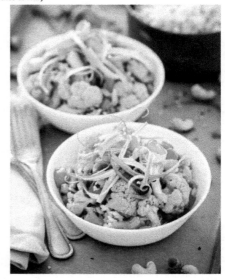

1. **To make the sauce** : Combine the water, tamari, vinegar, tomato paste, maple syrup, sriracha, and ginger in a cup or small bowl. Add the arrowroot and stir until combined. Set aside.

2. Heat the sesame oil in a large shallow saucepan or wok over medium heat. Add the red pepper flakes and stir constantly for about 2 minutes, making sure not to let the flakes burn. Add the onion and sauté until translucent. Add the cauliflower and liquid aminos, cover, and cook for 4 to 5 minutes, until heated through and the sauce is thickened. Add the garlic and bell pepper and cook, stirring occasionally, until the veggies are tender.

3. Add the cashews and the white parts of the green onions, then pour the sauce over the veggies. Cook for 3 to 4 minutes, stirring once or twice, until the sauce is thickened and heated through. Remove from the heat and add salt and pepper, if necessary. Serve over noodles or rice, garnished with the green onion strands. Keep any leftovers in an airtight container in the fridge for up to 4 days.

Creamy Spinach-Artichoke Pasta

SERVES 4

PREP TIME: **15 minutes** (not including time to make Pepita Parmesan)
ACTIVE TIME: **20 minutes**

One 12-ounce package frozen chopped spinach, thawed (see Tip)
1 pound penne or rigatoni pasta (gluten-free if necessary)
One 12-ounce vacuum-packed block extra firm silken tofu
1½ cups unsweetened nondairy milk (nut-free if necessary)
⅓ cup nutritional yeast
¼ cup vegan white wine
¼ cup lemon juice
3 tablespoons arrowroot powder
2 teaspoons garlic powder
2 teaspoons onion powder
¼ teaspoon cayenne pepper
1 tablespoon vegan butter
One 14- to 15-ounce can artichoke hearts, rinsed, drained, and quartered if whole
2 garlic cloves, minced
Salt and black pepper to taste
 Pepita Parmesan , optional

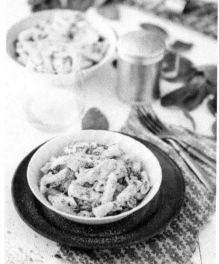

1. Place the spinach in a clean kitchen towel. Wrap the kitchen towel around the spinach and twist to squeeze out all the extra liquid. Set the spinach aside.

2. Bring a large pot of water to a boil, add a bit of salt, and add the pasta. Cook the pasta according to the package instructions until al dente. Drain and set the pasta aside.

3. While the pasta is cooking, combine the tofu, milk, nutritional yeast, wine, lemon juice, arrowroot, garlic powder, onion powder, and cayenne pepper in a blender and blend until smooth. Set aside.

4. Melt the butter in a large shallow saucepan over medium heat. Add the artichokes and cook, stirring occasionally, for 3 to 4 minutes, until they begin to brown. Add the minced garlic and spinach and cook until heated through. Add the pasta and tofu mixture and stir, cooking until heated through. Add salt and pepper, then remove from the heat. Serve topped with Pepita Parmesan (if using). Leftovers will keep in an airtight container in the fridge for up to 3 days.

TIP

▶ If you can't find a 12-ounce package frozen chopped spinach, 10 ounces will also work, or you can thaw 1 pound and leave a little bit out.

85

VEGAN SANDWICHES

HEARTY AND SATISFYING MEAT-FREE SANDWICHES

Fillet o' Chickpea Sandwich with Tartar Sauce Slaw

MAKES 6 SANDWICHES

PREP TIME: **25 minutes** (not including time to cook brown rice and make Basic Cashew Cheese Sauce)
ACTIVE TIME: **50 minutes**
INACTIVE TIME: **2 hours**

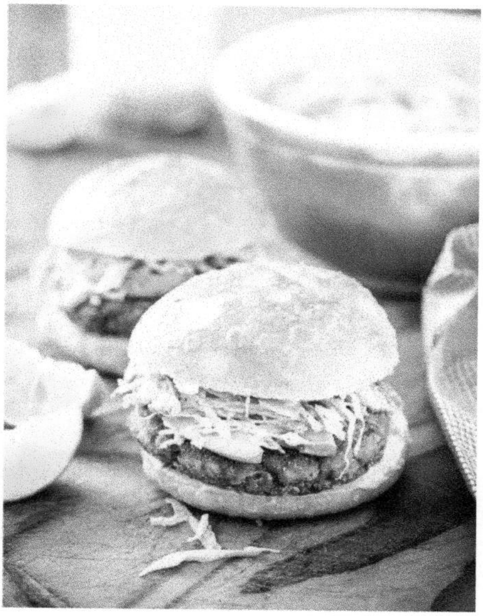

tartar sauce

½ cup raw cashews, soaked in warm water for 1 hour and drained, water reserved
¼ cup reserved soaking water
¼ cup vegan mayonnaise (soy-free if necessary)
¼ cup lemon juice
1 tablespoon caper brine
1 teaspoon dried dill

slaw

3 cups shredded cabbage
1 cup grated carrot

chickpea fillets

1½ cups cooked chickpeas (or one 15-ounce can, rinsed and drained)
1 tablespoon liquid aminos (use coconut aminos to be soy-free)
One 14- to 15-ounce can artichoke hearts, rinsed and drained
1 cup cooked brown rice
¼ cup + 1 tablespoon chickpea flour, plus more if needed
1 tablespoon Old Bay Seasoning
½ to 1 teaspoon kelp granules
½ teaspoon dried dill
Salt and black pepper to taste
1½ cups vegan bread crumbs (gluten-free if necessary)
Vegetable oil for pan-frying

sandwiches

Basic Cashew Cheese Sauce

6 vegan sandwich rolls or burger buns (gluten-free if necessary), split horizontally
Sliced avocado

1. **To make the tartar sauce** : Combine the tartar sauce ingredients in a food processor or blender and process until smooth.

2. **To make the slaw** : Combine the shredded cabbage and carrots in a large bowl and add ½ cup of the tartar sauce. Mix until fully combined and chill for at least 1 hour. Transfer the remaining tartar sauce to a small bowl and refrigerate until needed.

3. **To make the chickpea fillets** : Heat a large frying pan, preferably cast iron, over medium heat. Add the chickpeas and cook for a couple of minutes. Add the liquid aminos and cook for 5 to 7 minutes, stirring occasionally, until the liquid has been absorbed. Remove from the heat. Use a fork or pastry cutter to gently mash the chickpeas. You only have to mash them a bit; you still want them a little chunky.

4. Place the artichoke hearts in a food processor and pulse 5 to 7 times, until the artichokes are broken down into little pieces but not mushy.

5. Combine the chickpeas, artichokes, rice, and chickpea flour in a large bowl. Use your hands to mash the mixture until it's fully combined and will hold together when you squeeze it. If it doesn't hold together, add more chickpea flour by the tablespoon until it holds. Add the Old Bay, kelp granules to taste, the dill, salt, and pepper and mix until combined.

6. Line a baking sheet with parchment paper or a silicone baking mat. Line a plate with paper towels to drain the cooked fillets.

7. Pour the bread crumbs into a shallow bowl. Divide the chickpea mixture into six equal portions. One at a time, shape each into the fillet shape of your choice (round, square, rectangle), place in the bread crumbs, and gently flip until all sides are covered. Gently shake off the excess crumbs and place on the prepared baking sheet.

8. Heat a large frying pan over medium heat. Add oil until the bottom of the pan is thinly coated. Once the oil begins to shimmer, add 2 or 3 fillets. Cook for 2 to 3 minutes on each side, until both sides are golden. Transfer the fillets to the paper-towel-lined plate to drain the excess oil. Cover with a clean kitchen cloth to keep warm while you repeat with the remaining filets (adding more oil to the pan if necessary).

9. **To assemble each sandwich** : Spread cheese on the bottom half of a roll and spread tartar sauce on the top half. Place a fillet on top of the cheese sauce, then add some avocado slices, a pile of slaw, and cover with the top half of the roll. Serve immediately. If you plan to eat the sandwich later, store it in an airtight container and refrigerate for up 5 hours. Leftover fillets will keep in an airtight container in the fridge for 3 to 4 days.

The Portobello Philly Reuben

MAKES 4 SANDWICHES

PREP TIME: **15 minutes** (not including time to make Smoked Gouda Cheese Sauce)
ACTIVE TIME: **20 minutes** INACTIVE TIME: **10 minutes**

Russian dressing
⅓ cup vegan mayonnaise (soy-free if necessary)
1 tablespoon ketchup
1 tablespoon no-salt-added tomato paste
2 teaspoons red wine vinegar
1 teaspoon dried dill
½ teaspoon smoked paprika
2 to 3 tablespoons sweet pickle relish

sandwiches
4 portobello mushroom caps
Olive oil spray
2 tablespoons liquid aminos (or gluten-free tamari; use coconut aminos to be soy-free)
2 tablespoons vegan Worcestershire sauce (gluten-free and/or soy-free if necessary)
Black pepper to taste
4 vegan sandwich rolls (gluten-free if necessary), split horizontally
Smoked Gouda Cheese Sauce, Melty Variation
Loads of sauerkraut

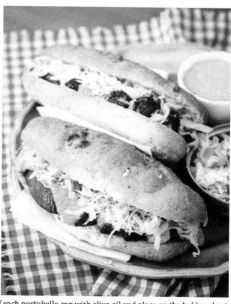

1. **To make the Russian dressing** : Stir together the mayonnaise, ketchup, tomato paste, vinegar, dill, and paprika in a small bowl. Add relish to taste. Chill until ready to use.

2. **To make the sandwiches** : Preheat the oven to 425°F. Line a baking sheet with parchment paper or a silicone baking mat. Lightly spray the top and bottom of each portobello cap with olive oil and place on the baking sheet gill side up.

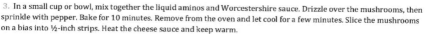

3. In a small cup or bowl, mix together the liquid aminos and Worcestershire sauce. Drizzle over the mushrooms, then sprinkle with pepper. Bake for 10 minutes. Remove from the oven and let cool for a few minutes. Slice the mushrooms on a bias into ½-inch strips. Heat the cheese sauce and keep warm.

4. Preheat the broiler. Arrange the rolls on the baking sheet, cut side up. Lay portobello strips on the bottom halves. Spread or drop cheese sauce on top of the mushrooms. Place under the broiler for 1 to 2 minutes, until the cheese is golden and the bread is toasted.

5. Add a pile of sauerkraut onto the cheesy half of each sandwich, then spread Russian dressing on the top half of each roll. Place the top half on top of the sandwich and serve immediately.

BBQ Pulled Jackfruit Sandwich

PREP TIME: **10 minutes** (not including time to make Creamy, Crunchy Coleslaw)
ACTIVE TIME: **20 minutes**
INACTIVE TIME: **20 minutes**

BBQ jackfruit

One 20-ounce can jackfruit (packed in brine or water, not syrup)
1 teaspoon olive oil
½ sweet onion, chopped
1 garlic clove, minced
½ teaspoon ground cumin
½ teaspoon smoked paprika
¾ cup vegan barbecue sauce (homemade or store-bought)
1 to 2 tablespoons sriracha
2 teaspoons arrowroot powder
Salt and black pepper to taste

sandwiches

4 vegan sandwich rolls or burger buns (gluten-free if necessary), split horizontally
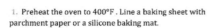 Creamy, Crunchy Coleslaw
Sliced avocado, optional

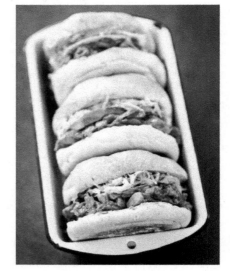

1. Preheat the oven to 400°F. Line a baking sheet with parchment paper or a silicone baking mat.

2. Rinse and drain the jackfruit. Use two forks or your fingers to pull it apart into shreds, so that it somewhat resembles pulled meat. It will fall apart even more when you cook it.

3. Heat the oil in a large shallow saucepan over medium heat. Add the onion and garlic and sauté until the onion is translucent. Add the jackfruit, cumin, and paprika and cook, stirring occasionally, for about 5 minutes. Add salt and pepper.

4. In a cup or small bowl, stir together the barbecue sauce, sriracha, and arrowroot powder. Add to the jackfruit. Cook for 1 minute.

5. Spread out the jackfruit on the prepared baking sheet. Bake for 20 minutes, stirring once halfway through, until sauce is thick and sticky.

6. **To assemble the sandwich** : Open a roll on a plate. Place avocado slices (if using) on the bottom half. Scoop a heap of the jackfruit on top, then top the jackfruit with a pile of coleslaw. Place the other half of the roll on top and serve immediately. Leftover jackfruit will keep in an airtight container in the fridge for 3 to 4 days.

The Avocado Melt

MAKES 2 SANDWICHES

PREP TIME: **15 minutes** (not including time to Basic Cashew Cheese Sauce)
ACTIVE TIME: **10 minutes**

4 bread slices (gluten-free if necessary)
Vegan butter (soy-free if necessary)
1 avocado, pitted, peeled, and sliced
Salt and black pepper to taste
½ batch Basic Cashew Cheese Sauce, _Melty Variation_ (see Tip)
Optional add-ins: _Quick Bacon Crumbles_ , _Pickled Red Cabbage & Onion Relish_ , sliced tomatoes, chopped green onions
Vegan mayonnaise (soy-free if necessary)

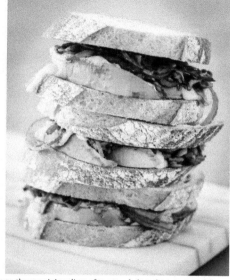

1. Preheat the broiler.

2. Toast the bread in a toaster on a medium setting—you don't want it to get too toasted. Lightly butter the toast. Spread out half of the avocado slices on each of two slices of toast. Place both on a baking sheet. Sprinkle salt and pepper over the avocado. Drizzle or dollop cheese sauce on top. Place the baking sheet under the broiler for about 2 minutes, until the cheese is lightly browned. Remove from the oven and top with your desired add-ins (if using). Spread mayonnaise on the remaining slices of toast and place them on top of the sandwiches. Serve immediately.

TIP

▶ Heat the cheese sauce right before you're ready to put the sandwiches in the oven.

Chickenless Salad Sandwich

MAKES 4 SANDWICHES

PREP TIME: **15 minutes**
ACTIVE TIME: **15 minutes** INACTIVE TIME: **1 hour + 50 minutes**

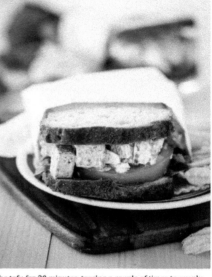

½ cup low-sodium "no-chicken" flavored vegetable broth (or regular low-sodium vegetable broth)
¼ cup liquid aminos (or gluten-free tamari; use coconut aminos to be soy-free)
1 teaspoon dried thyme
½ teaspoon dried marjoram
½ teaspoon garlic powder
½ teaspoon onion powder
½ teaspoon paprika
½ teaspoon liquid smoke
One 14-ounce block extra firm tofu, drained and pressed for 1 hour (see How to Press Tofu)
⅓ cup vegan mayonnaise
1 teaspoon Dijon mustard (gluten-free if necessary)
1 teaspoon dried dill
2 celery stalks, halved lengthwise and finely chopped
¼ small yellow onion, diced
Salt and black pepper to taste
Lettuce
Sliced tomato
8 vegan bread slices (or 4 vegan sandwich rolls; gluten-free if necessary)

1. Combine the broth, liquid aminos, thyme, marjoram, garlic powder, onion powder, paprika, and liquid smoke in an 8 × 8-inch baking dish. Slice the tofu into ½-inch cubes, add to the marinade, and toss until coated. Marinate the tofu for 20 minutes, tossing a couple of times to evenly distribute the marinade.

2. Preheat the oven to 350°F. Line a baking sheet with parchment paper or a silicone baking mat. Use a slotted spoon to scoop and spread the tofu onto the prepared baking sheet. Bake for 30 minutes, tossing once halfway through, until crisp and golden brown. Remove the tofu from the oven and let cool for about 5 minutes.

3. Combine the mayonnaise, mustard, and dill in a large bowl. Add the celery, onion, and tofu and stir until thoroughly combined. Season with salt and pepper. You can eat it right away or chill it before serving to allow the flavors to marry. The salad can be made up to 2 days before serving.

4. To assemble each sandwich, place some lettuce and sliced tomato on one bread slice (or the bottom half of a roll). Add a big pile of the salad and top with another slice of bread or the top of the roll. Serve immediately, or store the sandwiches in an airtight container in the fridge for up to 5 hours.

Lemongrass Tofu Banh Mi

MAKES 2 LARGE OR 4 SMALL SANDWICHES, WITH EXTRA SALAD

PREP TIME: **25 minutes**
ACTIVE TIME: **25 minutes**
INACTIVE TIME: **24 hours**

pickled carrot & daikon salad
1 cup julienned carrot
1 cup julienned daikon radish
1 small jalapeño, sliced
½ cup water
¼ cup rice vinegar
2 tablespoons agave syrup
¼ teaspoon salt

lemongrass tofu
One 14-ounce block extra firm tofu, drained and pressed
for at least 30 minutes (see How to Press Tofu)
4 lemongrass stalks, ends trimmed and outer leaves
discarded, roughly chopped
1 garlic clove, minced
2 tablespoons water
2 tablespoons gluten-free tamari
1 tablespoon lemon juice
1 teaspoon maple syrup
1 teaspoon sriracha
1 teaspoon liquid smoke
1 tablespoon coconut oil
2 tablespoons sesame seeds, optional

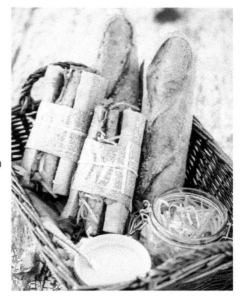

sriracha aïoli
½ cup vegan mayonnaise
1 or 2 garlic cloves, minced and pressed
2 tablespoons lemon juice
1 tablespoon sriracha

sandwiches
1 long vegan baguette (or 2 large or 4 small vegan sandwich rolls; gluten-free if necessary), split horizontally
1 cup thinly sliced cucumber
Chopped fresh cilantro
Sliced jalapeño
Chopped green onions (green and white parts)

1. A day prior to serving, **make the salad** : Combine the carrot and daikon with the jalapeño in a large jar or other airtight container. Stir together the water, vinegar, agave syrup, and salt in a large measuring cup. Pour the brine over the veggies and cover with a tight-fitting lid. Shake the container to fully mix everything together, then refrigerate for at least 1 day. It will keep for 2 weeks.

2. **To make the lemongrass tofu** : Chop the tofu in half both ways, making four rectangles. Combine the lemongrass, garlic, water, tamari, lemon juice, maple syrup, sriracha, and liquid smoke in a blender. Blend until smooth. If necessary, add more water by the tablespoon to thin it into a sauce. Pour into an 8 × 8-inch baking dish. Place the tofu rectangles in the baking dish and turn over so both sides are covered in the marinade. Let the tofu marinate for 20 minutes, flipping them once halfway through.

3. While the tofu is marinating, **make the aïoli** : Combine all the ingredients in a small cup or bowl, stirring until well mixed.

4. After the tofu has finished marinating, heat the coconut oil in a large frying pan, preferably cast iron, over medium heat. Add the tofu rectangles and cook for 2 to 3 minutes per side, until each side has a crispy, golden exterior. Drizzle half of the leftover marinade into the pan and cook the tofu for 1 minute more, or until the liquid has been absorbed. Flip the tofu, add the remaining marinade, and cook until the liquid has been absorbed. Add the sesame seeds and toss until coated. Remove from the heat.

5. Slice the rounded ends off the baguette, then cut it in half to make two large sandwiches or into four pieces for small sandwiches.

6. **To assemble each sandwich** : Spread aïoli on the bottom half of the bread. Lay a few cucumber slices on the aïoli, then place tofu on top of the cucumber slices. (If you're making two large sandwiches, use two pieces of tofu. If you're making four small sandwiches, just use one piece per sandwich.) Top the tofu with some carrot and daikon salad, cilantro, jalapeño, and green onions. Serve immediately. To eat the sandwich later, store it in an airtight container and refrigerate for up to 5 hours. Leftover tofu will keep in an airtight container in the fridge for 4 to 5 days.

VEGAN BAKING

VEGAN BAKED GOODS THAT YOU DON'T HAVE TO BE A HIPPIE TO LOVE

95

Blueberry-Banana Muffins

MAKES 12 MUFFINS

PREP TIME: **10 minutes**
ACTIVE TIME: **25 minutes**
INACTIVE TIME: **20 minutes**

¾ cup nondairy milk (nut-free and/or soy-free if necessary)
1 teaspoon apple cider vinegar
2 cups oat flour (certified gluten-free if necessary)
⅓ cup sweet white rice flour
1 tablespoon cornstarch (or arrowroot powder)
1 tablespoon baking powder
½ teaspoon ground cinnamon
½ teaspoon salt
2 ripe (very speckled) medium bananas, mashed
⅓ cup maple syrup
2 tablespoons coconut oil, melted
1 tablespoon flax meal
1 teaspoon vanilla extract
1 cup fresh blueberries (see Tip)
⅓ cup coconut sugar

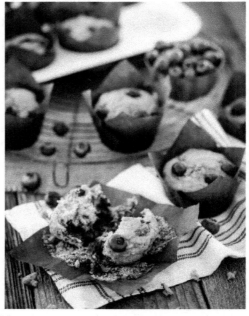

1. Preheat the oven to 350°F. Line a 12-cup muffin tin with paper or silicone liners.

2. Combine the milk and vinegar in a cup or small bowl. Set aside.

3. Combine the oat flour, rice flour, cornstarch, baking powder, cinnamon, and salt in a large bowl and whisk until thoroughly combined.

4. Combine the bananas, maple syrup, coconut oil, flax meal, and vanilla in a medium bowl and add the milk mixture. Stir until combined. Add the wet ingredients to the dry ingredients and stir together until combined. Fold in the blueberries and sugar.

5. Pour the batter into the muffin tin. Bake for 23 to 25 minutes, until the tops are golden and firm. Let the muffins cool in the tin for about 5 minutes before transferring to a cooling rack. Cool completely before serving. Leftovers will keep in the fridge or at room temperature for 3 to 4 days.

TIP

 You can use frozen blueberries instead of fresh, but to prevent them from bleeding, make sure to keep them in the freezer until just before you use them.

Chocolate Layer Cake

SERVES 12

PREP TIME: **15 minutes**
ACTIVE TIME: **40 minutes**
INACTIVE TIME: **60 minutes**

chocolate cake

Vegan cooking spray (or vegan butter; soy-free if necessary)
2¼ cups unsweetened vanilla nondairy milk (nut-free and/or soy-free if necessary)
3 tablespoons apple cider vinegar
3 cups white rice flour
1½ cups cocoa powder
¼ cup + 2 tablespoons oat flour (certified gluten-free if necessary)
¼ cup + 2 tablespoons coconut sugar
1 tablespoon baking powder
1 tablespoon baking soda
1½ teaspoons salt
1 cup maple syrup
12 tablespoons vegan butter (soy-free if necessary), melted
½ cup + 1 tablespoon aquafaba
1 tablespoon vanilla extract

frosting

1 cup vegan chocolate chips (or chunks)
3 cups pitted Medjool dates
1 cup unsweetened vanilla nondairy milk (nut-free and/or soy-free if necessary)
¼ cup cocoa powder
1 teaspoon vanilla extract
½ teaspoon salt
Vegan chocolate shavings, optional

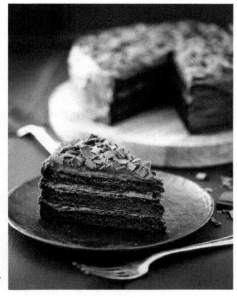

1. Preheat the oven to 350°F. Lightly spray three 9-inch cake pans with cooking spray or grease them with a bit of butter.

2. **To make the cake** : Combine the milk and vinegar in a medium bowl. Set aside.

3. Whisk together the rice flour, cocoa powder, oat flour, sugar, baking powder, baking soda, and salt in a large bowl.

4. Add the maple syrup, butter, aquafaba, and vanilla to the milk mixture and whisk until combined. Add the wet ingredients to the dry ingredients and stir until thoroughly combined and smooth.

5. Distribute the batter evenly among the three pans. Bake for 35 to 40 minutes, until a toothpick inserted into the center comes out clean. Let the layers cool in the pans for about 30 minutes. Run a knife around the inside edge of the cake pans and gently transfer the layers to cooling racks to let them cool completely.

6. Once the layers come out of the oven, **make the frosting** : Melt the chocolate chips in a double boiler or a heatproof bowl on top a pot of boiling water, stirring occasionally, until smooth. Remove from the heat. Combine the dates and milk in a food processor and process until smooth. Add the melted chocolate, cocoa powder, vanilla, and salt and process until smooth. Transfer the frosting to a jar and refrigerate for at least 30 minutes, or until ready to use.

7. Once the frosting has chilled and thickened, place one of the layers on a plate or serving dish. Using a thin silicone spatula or a butter knife, evenly spread a layer of frosting on top. Place another layer on top of the frosting. Evenly spread frosting on the top of the second layer, then top with the third layer. Spread the rest of the frosting evenly over the top and around the sides until the entire cake is covered. Top with chocolate shavings, if desired. Slice and serve. The cake will keep, covered, at room temperature or in the fridge for 3 to 4 days.

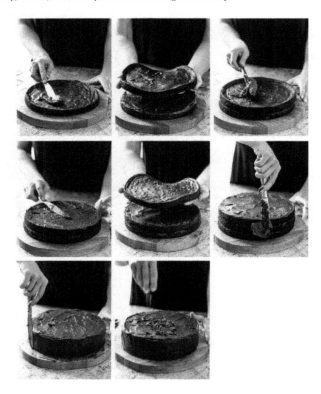

VARIATION

▶ To make 12 cupcakes, divide the quantity of the cake ingredients by three and the frosting ingredients by two. Line the cups of a 12-cup muffin tin with paper or silicone liners and distribute the batter evenly among the cups. Bake for 18 to 20 minutes, until a toothpick inserted into the center comes out almost clean. Let the cupcakes cool in the tin for 30 minutes before transferring them to the cooling rack. Cool completely before frosting.

TIP

▶ The frosted cake will gain moisture and firmness if refrigerated in an airtight container overnight.

Peanut Butter Oatmeal Cookies

MAKES 30 COOKIES

PREP TIME: **10 minutes**
ACTIVE TIME: **20 minutes**
INACTIVE TIME: **10 minutes**

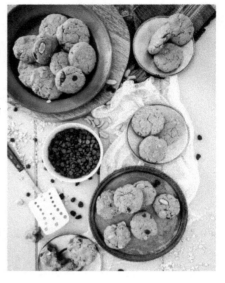

1 cup unbleached all-purpose flour (or gluten-free flour blend, soy-free if necessary)
1 cup rolled oats (certified gluten-free if necessary)
1 teaspoon baking soda
1 teaspoon ground cinnamon
½ teaspoon salt
½ teaspoon xanthan gum (exclude if using all-purpose flour or if your gluten-free blend includes it)
¼ teaspoon ground nutmeg
1 cup unsalted, unsweetened natural peanut butter
½ cup maple syrup
⅓ cup unsweetened applesauce (or mashed banana)
¼ cup coconut oil, melted
¼ cup coconut sugar, optional
1 teaspoon vanilla extract

Optional add-ins: ½ cup raisins, chopped peanuts, and/or vegan chocolate chips

1. Preheat the oven to 350°F. Line two baking sheets with parchment paper or silicone baking mats.

2. In a large bowl, whisk together the flour, oats, baking soda, cinnamon, salt, xanthan gum (if using), and nutmeg until fully incorporated.

3. In a medium bowl, combine the peanut butter, maple syrup, applesauce, coconut oil, coconut sugar (if using), and vanilla. Stir until combined.

4. Add the wet ingredients to the dry ingredients and stir until combined. If you're using add-ins, fold them in.

5. Scoop a heaping tablespoon of dough out of the bowl, roll it in your hands to make a perfect ball, and place it on the baking sheet. Repeat with the remaining dough, spacing the balls 1½ inches apart. Use your fingers to gently flatten each ball just a bit.

6. Bake for 10 to 12 minutes, until firm and slightly golden along the bottom. Let the cookies cool on the baking sheets for about 5 minutes before transferring them to a cooling rack. Cool completely before serving. The cookies will keep stored in an airtight container (in the fridge if the weather is warm) for 3 to 4 days.

Salted Vanilla Maple Blondies

MAKES 12 BARS

PREP TIME: **15 minutes**
ACTIVE TIME: **15 minutes** INACTIVE TIME: **35 minutes**

1½ cups oat flour (certified gluten-free if necessary)
¼ cup sweet white rice flour
¼ cup coconut sugar (or brown sugar)
2 tablespoons tapioca powder
½ teaspoon baking soda
½ teaspoon salt
½ cup cashew butter (see Tip)
½ cup maple syrup
½ cup unsweetened applesauce
1 tablespoon coconut oil, melted
1 tablespoon apple cider vinegar
Scrapings from inside 1 vanilla bean (or 1 teaspoon vanilla powder)
1 teaspoon vanilla extract
Flaked sea salt

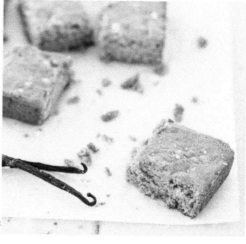

1. Preheat the oven to 350°F. Line an 8 × 8-inch baking dish with parchment paper. Let some hang over the edges, to make it easy to removed the blondies from the pan.

2. Whisk together the oat flour, rice flour, coconut sugar, tapioca powder, baking soda, and salt in a medium bowl.

3. Use a hand mixer to mix together the cashew butter, maple syrup, applesauce, and coconut oil in a large bowl. Stir in the vinegar, vanilla bean scrapings, and vanilla extract. Gradually stir the dry ingredients into the wet ingredients until well incorporated. Pour the batter into the prepared baking dish and lightly sprinkle sea salt flakes over the top.

4. Bake for 30 to 35 minutes, until the top is golden brown and firm and a toothpick inserted into the center comes out clean. Remove from the oven and let cool completely in the pan.

5. Once cool, use the parchment paper to lift the blondie out of the baking dish. Slice into 12 pieces. You can store the blondies in an airtight container at room temperature, but they'll hold their moisture longer when refrigerated. They'll keep for 3 to 4 days.

VARIATION

I'm sure I don't need to tell all you crazy chocoholics out there that these blondies are just *begging* for chocolate chips. Fold ½ cup vegan chocolate chips into the batter before transferring to the baking dish.

TIP

If you don't have cashew butter, soak 1 cup raw cashews in warm water for 1 hour. Drain and discard the soaking water. Place the cashews in a food processor and process until smooth. You can then add the maple syrup, applesauce, vinegar, vanilla bean scraping, and vanilla extract directly to the processor and process until smooth, rather than dirty up another bowl.

Pumpkin Chai Scones

MAKES 8 SCONES

PREP TIME: **15 minutes**
ACTIVE TIME: **30 minutes**
INACTIVE TIME: **30 minutes**

scones

½ cup unsweetened vanilla nondairy milk (nut-free and/or soy-free if necessary)
1 teaspoon apple cider vinegar
2 cups unbleached all-purpose flour (or gluten-free flour blend, soy-free if necessary)
⅓ cup coconut sugar (or brown sugar)
2 teaspoons baking powder
1 teaspoon baking soda
1 teaspoon ground cinnamon
1 teaspoon ground ginger
½ teaspoon ground cardamom
¼ teaspoon ground cloves
¼ teaspoon ground nutmeg
¼ teaspoon salt
¼ teaspoon xanthan gum (exclude if using all-purpose flour or if your gluten-free blend includes it)
8 tablespoons very cold vegan butter (soy-free if necessary)
½ cup pureed pumpkin (not pumpkin pie filling)
1 teaspoon vanilla extract
Oat flour (certified gluten-free if necessary) for dusting and kneading

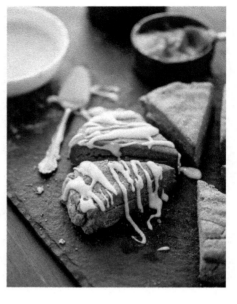

icing

½ cup powdered sugar (or xylitol)
1 tablespoon unsweetened vanilla nondairy milk (nut-free and/or soy-free if necessary)
Pinch of ground cinnamon

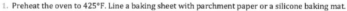

1. Preheat the oven to 425°F. Line a baking sheet with parchment paper or a silicone baking mat.

2. Combine the milk and vinegar in a medium bowl and set aside.

3. Combine the flour, coconut sugar, baking powder, baking soda, cinnamon, ginger, cardamom, cloves, nutmeg, salt, and xanthan gum (if using) in a large bowl. Whisk together until fully combined. Cut in the butter until all the pieces are smaller than your pinkie fingernail and the mixture has the texture of wet sand.

4. Add the pumpkin and vanilla to the milk mixture and stir until combined. Add the wet ingredients to the dry ingredients and stir until combined. The dough will be wet and sticky.

5. Generously flour your work surface with oat flour. Turn the dough out onto the surface and use your hands to scoop flour onto the ball of dough until all sides are coated. Gently flatten the dough a bit, then fold it over on top of itself. It's okay if it tears, just patch it up the best you can. Flatten the dough again, then sprinkle some more flour on top and

spread it out so that the top is coated. Fold it over on itself again. Repeat flouring and folding about five more times, until the dough is still soft and pliable and doesn't fall apart when folded, but don't overdo it to the point where the dough gets tough.

6. Shape the dough into an 8-inch circle. Slice into eight equal-size triangles. Place them on the prepared baking sheet. Bake for 15 to 20 minutes, until lightly browned and firm. Let the scones cool on the pan for about 10 minutes before

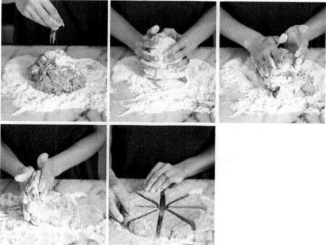

transferring them to a cooling rack to cool completely.

7. While the scones are cooling, **make the icing:** Combine all the ingredients in a small bowl and whisk with a fork until smooth.

8. Once the scones are cool, drizzle the icing over the tops. The scones will keep in an airtight container at room temperature for 2 to 3 days.

TIP

▶ For those who are patience deficient, just let the scones cool for 10 minutes, skip the icing, and enjoy right away.

Strawberry-Peach Crisp with Vanilla Whipped Cream

SERVES 8

PREP TIME: **20 minutes** (not including time to chill coconut cream)
ACTIVE TIME: **20 minutes**
INACTIVE TIME: **30 minutes**

filling

Vegan cooking spray (soy-free if necessary)
1 pound strawberries, hulled and quartered
3 medium peaches, pitted and thinly sliced
3 tablespoons coconut sugar (or brown sugar)
2 tablespoons lemon juice
1 tablespoon arrowroot powder
1 teaspoon grated fresh ginger

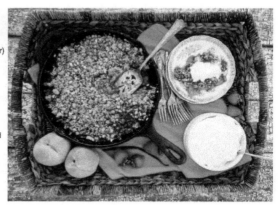

streusel

¾ cup oat flour (certified gluten-free if necessary)
½ cup corn flour (see _Flour Power_ ; certified gluten-free if necessary)
¼ cup brown rice flour
8 tablespoons cold vegan butter (soy-free if necessary)
½ cup rolled oats (certified gluten-free if necessary)
½ cup coconut sugar (or brown sugar)
½ teaspoon salt
½ teaspoon ground cinnamon
Scrapings from inside 1 vanilla bean, optional

vanilla whipped cream

One 14.5-ounce can unsweetened coconut cream (or full-fat coconut milk)
1 tablespoon powdered sugar (or xylitol)
½ teaspoon vanilla extract

1. The day before you plan to serve, refrigerate the can of coconut cream.

2. Preheat the oven to 400°F . Lightly spray a 10-inch cake pan, pie pan, or cast-iron skillet with cooking spray.

3. **To make the filling** : Combine the strawberries, peaches, coconut sugar, lemon juice, arrowroot, and ginger in a large bowl and stir until combined. Pour into the prepared baking dish.

4. **To make the streusel** : Whisk together the oat flour, corn flour, and rice flour. Cut in the butter until no piece is larger than your pinkie fingernail and the mixture has the texture of wet sand. Stir in the oats, sugar, salt, cinnamon, and vanilla bean scrapings (if using), just until evenly mixed. You want it to be clumpy but evenly distributed. Evenly spread the streusel over the fruit. Bake for 30 minutes, or until the topping is crispy and golden. Remove from the oven and let rest for 5 to 10 minutes before serving.

5. While the crisp is cooling, **make the whipped cream** : Carefully spoon the solid coconut cream into a large bowl, leaving the coconut water in the can (which you can totally keep to use for something else). Add the powdered sugar and vanilla to the cream and, using a hand mixer (fitted with a whisk attachment, if possible), mix on high speed until it has the texture of whipped cream. Transfer the bowl to the refrigerator until ready to serve.

6. Serve each helping of crisp topped with a dollop of whipped cream. Both the crisp and the whipped cream will keep in airtight containers in the fridge for 2 to 3 days.

VARIATION

▷ Strawberries and peaches not in season? Try using different pairings of fruit, such as cranberries and persimmons, apples and pears, or blueberries and mango. Just try to replace with similar quantities as much as possible, although if you get a little more or a little less, it's not going to hurt the final product.

VEGAN COMFORT FOOD

HEARTY, SHOW-STOPPING, MADE-OVER CLASSICS TO APPEASE EVEN THE LOUDEST NAYSAYERS

106

Hash Brown Casserole (aka Company Potatoes)

SERVES 6 TO 8

PREP TIME: **25 minutes** (not including time to make Cream of Mushroom Soup)
ACTIVE TIME: **5 minutes**
INACTIVE TIME: **35 minutes**

Olive oil spray
Cream of Mushroom Soup
¾ cup plain coconut yogurt (or soy yogurt; preferably unsweetened)
½ cup nutritional yeast
¾ cup sauerkraut
½ cup chopped yellow onion
One 20-ounce package frozen hash browns, thawed
3½ cups vegan cornflakes (certified gluten-free if necessary)
4 tablespoons vegan butter (soy-free if necessary), melted

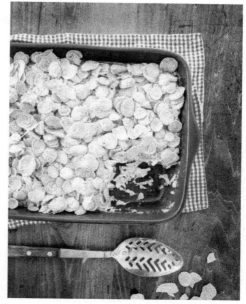

1. Preheat the oven to 350°F. Lightly spray a 9 × 13-inch baking dish with olive oil.

2. In a large bowl, stir together the soup, yogurt, and nutritional yeast. Stir in the sauerkraut, onion, and hash browns. Spread out the mixture in the prepared baking dish. Bake for 15 minutes.

3. While the casserole is baking, combine the cornflakes and melted butter in a medium bowl. After the casserole has baked for 15 minutes, spread the cornflakes over the top and return to the oven. Bake for 15 minutes more, or until the casserole is bubbly and the cornflakes are crispy and golden. Remove from the oven and let rest for 5 minutes before serving. Leftovers will keep in an airtight container in the fridge for up to 4 days.

Roasted Carrot & Wild Mushroom Ragout

SERVES 4

PREP TIME: **30 minutes** (not including time to make polenta)
ACTIVE TIME: **40 minutes**

8 large carrots, peeled and chopped into 1-inch pieces
Olive oil spray
1 teaspoon dried thyme
1 teaspoon dried parsley
Salt and black pepper to taste
3 cups water
2 ounces dried mushrooms (porcini or a mixed variety)
2 tablespoons vegan butter (soy-free if necessary)
½ red onion, chopped
2 garlic cloves, minced
1 tablespoon chopped fresh rosemary
1 tablespoon chopped fresh thyme
8 ounces button mushrooms (or cremini mushrooms), halved
8 ounces wild mushrooms (shiitake, chanterelle, oyster, morel, lobster, etc.; see Tip), sliced
2 tablespoons oat flour (certified gluten-free if necessary)
½ cup vegan red wine
3 tablespoons lemon juice
Cooked polenta or other grain or pasta
Chopped fresh parsley, optional

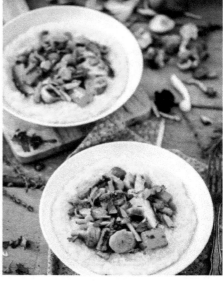

1. Preheat the oven to 425°F (220°C). Line a baking sheet with parchment paper or a silicone baking mat. Spread out the carrots on the sheet and lightly spray with olive oil. Sprinkle with the dried thyme, dried parsley, and salt and pepper. Toss to coat. Roast for 25 minutes, or until caramelized and tender. Set aside until ready to use.

2. Once the carrots are in the oven, bring the water to a boil in a medium pot, then remove from the heat. Add the dried mushrooms and set aside.

3. Melt the butter in a large shallow saucepan over medium heat. Add the onion and sauté until translucent. Add the garlic, rosemary, and fresh thyme and cook until fragrant, about 2 minutes. Add the button and wild mushrooms. Use a slotted spoon to scoop the rehydrated mushrooms from the water into the pan (do not discard the water). Cook for 8 to 10 minutes, stirring occasionally, until the mushrooms are tender but still hold their shape.

4. Add the oat flour and cook, stirring constantly, until the flour is fully incorporated. Add the wine and cook, stirring frequently, until the liquid has reduced. Add ½ cup of the reserved mushroom soaking water, bring to a boil, then reduce to a simmer. Cook for about 5 minutes, until most of the liquid has been absorbed.

5. Add the carrots, lemon juice, salt, and pepper and remove from the heat. Serve over creamy polenta, garnished with fresh parsley, if desired. Leftovers will keep in an airtight container in the fridge for 2 to 3 days.

Sweet Potato Shepherd's Pie

SERVES 6

PREP TIME: **15 minutes** (not including time
to make Pepita Parmesan)
ACTIVE TIME: **35 minutes**
INACTIVE TIME: **15 minutes**

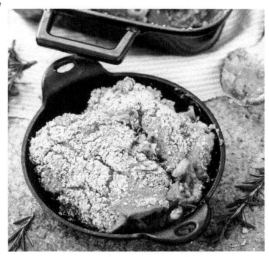

Olive oil spray

topping

2 pounds sweet potatoes or yams, peeled and
chopped
2 tablespoons unsweetened nondairy milk (nut-
free and/or soy-free if necessary)
2 tablespoons olive oil
1 tablespoon nutritional yeast, optional
½ teaspoon garlic powder
Salt and black pepper to taste
Pepita Parmesan
Chopped fresh rosemary

filling

1 teaspoon olive oil
1 red onion, diced
2 garlic cloves, minced
2 large carrots, peeled and chopped
3 celery stalks, chopped
3 cups cooked great Northern beans (or two 15-ounce cans), rinsed and drained)
8 ounces cremini mushrooms (or button mushrooms), sliced
1 tablespoon chopped fresh rosemary
1 tablespoon chopped fresh thyme
½ cup low-sodium vegetable broth
2 tablespoons liquid aminos (or gluten-free tamari; use coconut aminos to be soy-free)
2 tablespoons no-salt-added tomato paste
¼ cup chopped sun-dried tomatoes (rehydrated in water and drained, if necessary)
¼ cup chopped pitted green olives
1 tablespoon lemon juice
Salt and black pepper to taste

1. Preheat the oven to 400°F . Lightly spray an 8-inch square or 10-inch round baking dish with olive oil. Alternatively, if you have a shallow Dutch oven or large cast-iron skillet, you can use that to cook the filling, then bake the casserole.

2. **To make the topping** : Place the sweet potatoes in a medium pot and cover with water. Bring to a boil and cook for 8 to 10 minutes, until easily pierced with a fork. Remove from the heat and drain. Add the milk, olive oil, nutritional yeast (if using), and garlic powder and mash until smooth. Alternatively, you can use a hand mixer or food processor. Once smooth, add salt and pepper.

3. While the sweet potatoes are boiling, **make the filling** : Heat the olive oil in a large, shallow saucepan that can go into the oven (or a Dutch oven or cast-iron skillet) over medium heat. Add the onion and garlic and sauté for 2 to 3 minutes, until the onion just becomes translucent. Add the carrots and celery and cook for another 3 minutes. Add the beans, mushrooms, rosemary, and thyme. Cook for about 5 minutes, stirring occasionally.

4. Combine the broth, liquid aminos, and tomato paste in a cup or small bowl and stir until combined. Add to the vegetables with the sun-dried tomatoes and olives and cook for about 5 minutes more. Remove from the heat and add the lemon juice, salt, and pepper.

5. Pour the filling into the prepared pan (or leave it in the Dutch oven). Spread the mashed sweet potato over the top. Sprinkle with the Pepita Parmesan and rosemary. Bake for about 15 minutes, until the top is crispy and golden. Serve immediately. Leftovers will keep in an airtight container in the fridge for up to 4 days.

Lasagna Soup

SERVES 6

PREP TIME: **20 minutes** (not including time to make Herbed Macadamia Ricotta)
ACTIVE TIME: **35 minutes**

1 teaspoon olive oil
1 yellow onion, diced
3 garlic cloves, minced
1½ cups cooked chickpeas (or one 15-ounce can, rinsed and drained)
8 ounces cremini mushrooms (or button mushrooms), sliced
1 medium zucchini, sliced
1 medium yellow squash, sliced
1 tablespoon dried basil
2 teaspoons dried oregano
1 teaspoon dried parsley
Pinch of cayenne pepper
One 15-ounce can no-salt-added tomato sauce
One 15-ounce can no-salt-added crushed tomatoes
1 quart low-sodium vegetable broth
12 ounces lasagna noodles (gluten-free if necessary), broken in half
3 tablespoons nutritional yeast, optional
1 tablespoon lemon juice
Salt and black pepper to taste
3 cups loosely packed chopped fresh spinach
1 cup loosely packed chopped fresh basil
Herbed Macadamia Ricotta

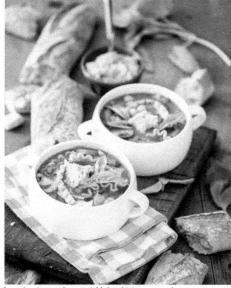

1. Bring a large pot of water to a boil.

2. Heat the olive oil in another large pot over medium heat. Add the onion and garlic and sauté until the onion is translucent. Add the chickpeas, mushrooms, zucchini, yellow squash, dried basil, oregano, parsley, and cayenne pepper and cook for about 5 minutes, stirring occasionally, until the vegetables are just becoming tender. Add the tomato sauce, tomatoes, and broth. Bring to a boil, then reduce to a simmer and cook for about 10 minutes.

3. While the soup is simmering, cook the lasagna noodles according to the package instructions until al dente. Drain the noodles and add to the soup. Stir in the nutritional yeast (if using), lemon juice, salt, and pepper. Add the spinach and fresh basil and remove from the heat. Serve immediately, topped with a dollop of ricotta. Leftovers will keep in an airtight container in the fridge for 3 to 4 days.

TIP

 If you let the soup simmer for too long after adding the noodles, the noodles will absorb more of the liquid and may break apart into smaller pieces. If you have leftovers, you may have to add more liquid when reheating.

Cauliflower Parmigiana

SERVES 4

PREP TIME: **30 minutes** (not including time to make Sun-Dried Tomato Marinara Sauce and Basic Cashew Cheese Sauce)

ACTIVE TIME: **20 minutes**

INACTIVE TIME: **40 minutes**

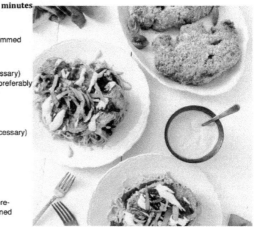

2 large heads cauliflower (3 to 4 pounds), leaves trimmed

coating
½ cup unsweetened nondairy milk (soy-free if necessary)
3 tablespoons plain coconut yogurt (or soy yogurt; preferably unsweetened)
1 teaspoon onion powder
1 teaspoon garlic powder
½ teaspoon smoked paprika
1 cup vegan panko bread crumbs (gluten-free if necessary)
½ cup oat flour (certified gluten-free if necessary)
¼ cup nutritional yeast
1 teaspoon dried basil
1 teaspoon dried oregano
Salt and black pepper to taste
Olive oil spray
3 cups Sun-Dried Tomato Marinara Sauce (or store-bought vegan marinara sauce of your choice), warmed
 Basic Cashew Cheese Sauce
½ cup chopped fresh basil

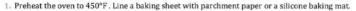

1. Preheat the oven to 450°F . Line a baking sheet with parchment paper or a silicone baking mat.

2. On a cutting board, hold one cauliflower upright and cut two 1½-inch-thick slices from the center of the head (without removing the core/base of the cauliflower). Repeat with the second head, so that you have four large slices. You can save the remaining cauliflower to use in other recipes, such as the Cream of Mushroom Soup .

3. In a wide, shallow bowl, combine the milk, yogurt, onion powder, garlic powder, and paprika. In a second wide, shallow bowl, combine the bread crumbs, oat flour, nutritional yeast, dried basil, oregano, salt, and pepper.

4. One at a time, place a cauliflower steak in the milk mixture, flipping it to fully coat (use a spoon to drizzle the liquid over the steak to coat it fully, if necessary). Transfer the steak to the bread crumbs, gently flipping until coated. Pat the bread crumbs onto the steak as needed. Place the steak on the prepared baking sheet. Once you've prepared each steak, you can coat the remaining cauliflower slices, if serving.

5. Spray the tops of the steaks liberally with olive oil. Bake for 20 minutes. Remove from the oven, gently flip each steak, and spray with olive oil again. Return to the oven and bake for 20 minutes more, or until golden and crispy.

6. To serve, scoop some marinara sauce onto each plate. Place a steak on top (along with a couple of other smaller pieces, if serving them). Drizzle with cheese sauce and sprinkle with fresh basil.

112

Brownie Ice Cream Sandwiches

MAKES 8 SANDWICHES

PREP TIME: **15 minutes** (not including time to make
Vanilla Ice Cream)
ACTIVE TIME: **25 minutes** INACTIVE TIME: **2½ hours**

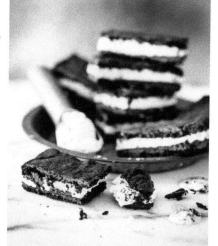

1 cup unbleached all-purpose flour (or gluten-free flour blend, soy-free
if necessary)
3 tablespoons Dutch-process cocoa powder
1 teaspoon baking powder
½ teaspoon baking soda
½ teaspoon xanthan gum (exclude if using all-purpose flour or if your
gluten-free blend includes it)
½ teaspoon salt
1 cup vegan dark chocolate chunks (or chips)
4 tablespoons vegan butter (soy-free if necessary)
½ cup coconut sugar (or brown sugar)
½ cup unsweetened applesauce
2 tablespoons aquafaba
1 teaspoon vanilla extract

Vanilla Ice Cream ; or 1½ pints store-bought vegan vanilla ice cream)

1. Preheat the oven to 350°F. Line two 8 × 8-inch baking dishes
with parchment paper. If you have them, use small binder clips to
clip the parchment paper to the edges of the dishes. This will keep
the paper from sliding when you spread the batter. Set the baking
dishes aside.

2. In a medium bowl, whisk together the flour, cocoa, baking powder, baking soda, xanthan gum (if using), and salt.

3. Melt the chocolate with the butter in a double boiler or a heatproof bowl on top of a pot of boiling water, stirring occasionally,
until smooth. Remove from the heat. Add the sugar, applesauce, aquafaba, and vanilla. Gradually stir the dry ingredients into the
wet ingredients.

4. Divide the batter between the two baking dishes and spread until smooth and even. The batter may be difficult to spread, so if
you need to, you can place a sheet of plastic wrap over the batter and use your hand to push or spread it. Bake for 25 to 30
minutes, until set and the edges are pulling away from the pan slightly. Remove from the oven and let cool for 1 to 2 hours.

5. Remove the ice cream from the freezer to soften for about 15 minutes before you plan to use it. Spread ice cream on top of the
brownie layer in one pan. Create an even layer that's ½ to 1 inch thick. (To spread it more easily, place a sheet of plastic wrap over
the ice cream and use your fingers to pat it down.)

6. Use the parchment paper to carefully lift the other brownie layer from the second dish and place it on top of the ice cream.
Gently press down to compress the sandwiches. Cover the pan and freeze for 30 to 60 minutes, until the ice cream is solid again.

7. Remove the pan from the freezer. Use the parchment paper to lift the big sandwich from the pan and place it on a flat surface,
such as a cutting board. Use a knife, cookie cutter, or biscuit cutter to cut out your desired sandwich shapes. If using a cookie or
biscuit cutter, you will have to gently push from the bottom, underneath the parchment paper, to get the sandwiches to pop up.
Place the sandwiches in an airtight container. Freeze until ready to serve, or for up to 1 month.

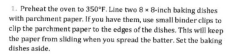

VEGAN FOR PICKY EATERS

ADAPTABLE MEALS THAT EVEN THE PICKIEST EATERS CAN ENJOY WITH THE REST OF YOU

IN THIS CHAPTER

Artichoke-Kale Hummus

BLT Summer Rolls with Avocado

Perfect Roasted Potatoes

Cauliflower Alfredo Baked Ziti

Creamy Roasted Garlic-Tomato Soup with Grilled Cheese Croutons

Chocolate-Peanut Butter Truffles

115

Artichoke-Kale Hummus

SERVES 8 TO 12

PREP TIME: **5 minutes**
ACTIVE TIME: **15 minutes**

3 cups cooked chickpeas (or two 15-ounce cans, rinsed and drained)
¼ cup lemon juice
3 tablespoons tahini (gluten-free if necessary)
3 garlic cloves
1 teaspoon ground cumin
1 teaspoon onion powder
¼ teaspoon cayenne pepper
Salt and black pepper to taste
3 cups packed chopped kale
One 14- to 15-ounce can artichoke hearts, rinsed, drained, and quartered if whole
Bread or crackers (gluten-free if necessary)

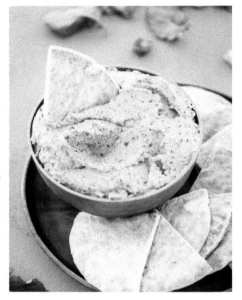

1. Combine the chickpeas, lemon juice, tahini, garlic, cumin, onion powder, and cayenne in a food processor and process until smooth. Taste and add salt and pepper as needed. If the dip is too thick, add water by the tablespoon until it reaches your desired thickness.

2. Add the kale and artichoke hearts and pulse until fully incorporated but still chunky. Serve immediately with bread or crackers or refrigerate until ready to use. Leftovers will keep in an airtight container in the fridge for 1 to 2 days.

VARIATIONS

▶ For those who hate hummus (*Who hates hummus?*), switch out the chickpeas with white beans and replace the tahini with olive oil.

▶ For kale haters, switch out the kale for spinach, chard, or collard greens. For those who hate greens altogether, they can be left out completely.

BLT Summer Rolls with Avocado

MAKES 8 ROLLS

PREP TIME: 15 minutes (not including time to make Quick Bacon Crumbles and Avocado Ranch Dressing or Lemon Dill Aïoli)
ACTIVE TIME: 25 minutes

Quick Bacon Crumbles (or 10 oz vegan bacon of your choice)
1 small head romaine lettuce, separated into leaves, each leaf chopped in half widthwise
2 to 3 Roma tomatoes, seeded and thinly sliced lengthwise
1 avocado, pitted, peeled, and sliced, optional
Eight 8-inch sheets rice paper (see Tip)
Avocado Ranch Dressing or Lemon Dill Aïoli

1. Fill a large bowl with warm water. Make sure you have a clean surface to prepare the rolls on.

2. Dip a sheet of rice paper into the water, making sure to get it completely wet but removing it quickly before it gets too soft. Lay the paper on the clean surface, then lay a few pieces of lettuce on the center of the paper, going from side to side and leaving about an inch of space around the perimeter. Add a few slices of tomato, a few slices of avocado (if using), and a few spoonfuls of the bacon crumbles (or 2 or 3 slices if you're using a sliced variety).

3. Fold the left and right sides of the paper over the filling. Take the edge of the paper closest to you and fold it completely over the filling while using your fingers to tuck the filling in. Continue rolling until the roll is sealed. Repeat with the remaining ingredients. Serve immediately with the Avocado Ranch Dressing or Lemon Dill Aïoli. These rolls are best enjoyed right after they're made but will keep in an airtight container in the fridge for 5 or 6 hours.

VARIATIONS

▷ For those who aren't fond of avocado, you can leave it out, and switch out the Avocado Ranch Dressing with a regular vegan ranch dressing, or use the Lemon Dill Aïoli.

▷ If your family isn't into summer rolls, just pile all the ingredients between two slices of bread for a sandwich. You won't get any complaints.

TIP

▷ Rice paper sheets that are 6 inches in diameter will be too small.

Perfect Roasted Potatoes

SERVES 4 TO 6

PREP TIME: **10 minutes**
ACTIVE TIME: **10 minutes**
INACTIVE TIME: **40 minutes**

Olive oil spray or vegan cooking spray (soy-free if necessary)
2 pounds Yukon gold potatoes, peeled and chopped into 1-inch cubes
4 tablespoons vegan butter (soy-free if necessary), melted (or ¼ cup olive oil)
2 teaspoons garlic powder
2 teaspoons dried thyme or rosemary

Salt and black pepper to taste

1. Preheat the oven to 400°F. Lightly spray two baking sheets with olive oil.

2. Place the potatoes in a medium pot and cover them with water. Bring to a boil and cook for 5 to 6 minutes, until tender. Drain.

3. Spread out the potatoes on the baking sheets. Use a spatula to gently smash each one just a little bit. Pour the butter over the potatoes. Sprinkle the garlic powder, thyme, salt, and pepper on top. Toss to coat, then spread them out again, making sure that the pieces aren't touching. Bake for 40 minutes, flipping them halfway through. Serve immediately. Leftovers will keep in an airtight container in the fridge for 2 to 3 days.

VARIATION

▷ Feel free to try other seasonings if garlic powder, thyme, or rosemary don't float your boat.

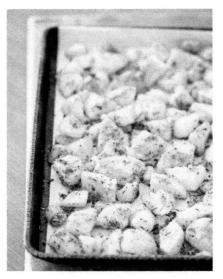

Cauliflower Alfredo Baked Ziti

SERVES 6 TO 8

PREP TIME: **10 minutes** (not including time to make Pepita Parmesan)
ACTIVE TIME: **30 minutes**
INACTIVE TIME: **50 minutes**

Olive oil spray or vegan cooking spray (soy-free if necessary)
1 large (1½- to 2-pound) head cauliflower, broken into florets
3 cups low-sodium vegetable broth
1 pound ziti or penne pasta (gluten-free if necessary)
1 cup raw cashews, soaked in warm water for at least 30 minutes and drained, water discarded
2 cups unsweetened nondairy milk (soy-free if necessary)
¼ cup nutritional yeast
¼ cup vegan white wine
3 tablespoons olive oil
3 tablespoons lemon juice
2 teaspoons white soy miso (or chickpea miso)
2 teaspoons onion powder
2 teaspoons garlic powder
¼ teaspoon ground nutmeg
Salt and black pepper to taste
Pepita Parmesan

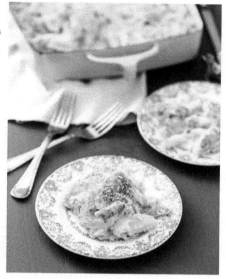

1. Preheat the oven to 350°F. Lightly spray a 9 × 13-inch baking dish with olive oil. Bring a large pot of water to a boil.

2. Combine the cauliflower and broth in a medium pot, cover, and bring to a boil. Reduce to a simmer, cover again, and simmer for 10 minutes, or until the cauliflower is soft. Remove from the heat.

3. Cook the pasta according to the package instructions until al dente. Drain. Set aside in a large bowl.

4. While the pasta is cooking, use a slotted spoon to scoop the cauliflower into a blender. (You can save the broth for another use.) Add the cashews, milk, nutritional yeast, wine, oil, lemon juice, miso, onion powder, garlic powder, nutmeg, salt, and pepper. Blend until smooth.

5. Add the sauce to the pasta. Stir until combined, then pour into the prepared baking dish. Sprinkle the Pepita Parmesan over the top and bake for 20 minutes. Serve immediately. Leftovers will keep in an airtight container in the fridge for up to 4 days.

VARIATION

▷ To add some flavor or texture, try adding sautéed mushrooms, caramelized onions, steamed broccoli, or cooked greens.

119

Creamy Roasted Garlic–Tomato Soup with Grilled Cheese Croutons

SERVES 4

PREP TIME: **20 minutes** (not including time to make Basic Cashew Cheese Sauce)
ACTIVE TIME: **45 minutes**
INACTIVE TIME: **40 minutes**

soup

3 to 4 pounds Roma tomatoes, halved lengthwise
1 teaspoon olive oil, plus more for roasting
Salt and black pepper to taste
1 small garlic head (see Variation)
1 sweet onion, diced
One 6-ounce can no-salt-added tomato paste
2 tablespoons coconut sugar (or brown sugar)
2 tablespoons white wine vinegar
2 teaspoons dried basil
1 teaspoon dried oregano
3 cups low-sodium vegetable broth
½ cup unsweetened nondairy milk (soy-free if necessary)
1 tablespoon nutritional yeast, optional

2 to 3 tablespoons chopped fresh basil, optional

croutons

4 vegan sandwich bread slices (gluten-free if necessary)
Basic Cashew Cheese Sauce, Melty Variation

Vegan butter (soy-free if necessary)

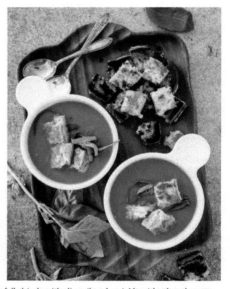

1. Preheat the oven to 400°F . Line one or two baking sheets with parchment paper or silicone baking mats. Spread out the tomato halves on the baking sheet(s), cut side up. Drizzle with olive oil and sprinkle with salt and pepper.

2. Trim the top off the head of garlic so that all the

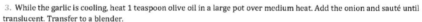

cloves are exposed. Place the head on a sheet of aluminum foil, drizzle with olive oil, and sprinkle with salt and pepper. Wrap the foil around the head so that it's completely enclosed. Roast the garlic and the tomatoes for about 40 minutes, until the garlic is soft and the tomatoes slightly charred. Remove from the oven. Unwrap the garlic so it can cool. Set the tomatoes aside.

3. While the garlic is cooling, heat 1 teaspoon olive oil in a large pot over medium heat. Add the onion and sauté until translucent. Transfer to a blender.

4. Once the garlic is cool to the touch, squeeze each clove over a small plate or bowl so that the garlic pops out. Transfer all the garlic to the blender along with the onions, roasted tomatoes, tomato paste, sugar, vinegar, dried basil, and oregano. Blend until smooth.

5. Combine the tomato mixture and broth in the large pot and bring to a boil. Reduce to a simmer and cook for about 15 minutes, stirring occasionally, until heated through and slightly thickened. Stir in the milk and nutritional yeast (if using) and cook for another 5 minutes. Reduce the heat to low and cover to keep the soup warm.

6. While the soup is simmering, **make the croutons** : Lay out 2 slices of bread, spread them with cheese, and top each with another slice of bread. Spread butter on the outsides of each sandwich. Heat a frying pan, preferably cast iron, over medium heat. Place both sandwiches in the pan and cook for 2 to 3 minutes per side, until each side is crispy and golden. Remove from the heat and cut each sandwich into six squares.

7. Spoon the soup into bowls and top each serving with a sprinkle of fresh basil (if using) and 3 or 4 grilled cheese croutons (or serve them on the side and add them as you eat). Serve immediately. Leftover soup will keep in an airtight container in the fridge for 3 to 4 days.

VARIATION

▶ If your family doesn't care for garlic, you can totally leave it out altogether.

Chocolate–Peanut Butter Truffles

MAKES 10 TO 12 TRUFFLES

PREP TIME: **5 minutes**
ACTIVE TIME: **20 minutes**
INACTIVE TIME: **55 minutes**

½ cup unsalted, unsweetened natural peanut butter
¼ cup oat flour (certified gluten-free if necessary)
2½ tablespoons powdered sugar (or xylitol)
Pinch of salt (exclude if using salted peanut butter)
1 cup vegan chocolate chips (or chopped vegan chocolate)
1 teaspoon coconut oil
Chopped peanuts, optional
Flaked sea salt, optional

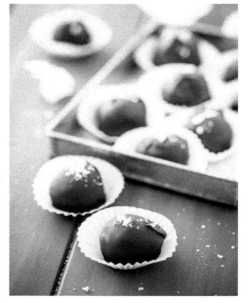

1. In a medium bowl, use a fork to stir together the peanut butter, oat flour, sugar, and salt (if using). Place the bowl in the freezer and leave it for 20 minutes, until firm.

2. Line a baking sheet with parchment paper or a silicone baking mat. Remove the peanut butter mixture from the freezer. Scoop up 1 tablespoon and use your hands to roll it into a ball. Place the ball on the prepared baking sheet. Repeat with the remaining peanut butter mixture. Place the sheet in the freezer to chill while you melt the chocolate, or for at least 15 minutes. If you don't plan on coating them with chocolate until later, just put the sheet in the refrigerator for at least 30 minutes.

3. Melt the chocolate with the coconut oil in a double boiler or heatproof bowl on top of a pot of boiling water, stirring frequently, until completely smooth. Remove from the heat.

4. Remove the peanut butter balls from the freezer. Use a fork to scoop up a ball and dunk it in the melted chocolate. Roll it around to cover it completely, then use the spoon to lift it out and drain off the excess chocolate. Place the truffle back on the baking sheet. Repeat with the remaining balls. Sprinkle the tops with chopped peanuts and/or flaked sea salt (if using).

5. Return the baking sheet to the refrigerator and chill until completely set, 15 to 20 minutes, or until ready to serve. The truffles will keep in an airtight container in the fridge for 4 to 5 days.

TIP

▶ If your peanut butter is very runny, add an additional 1 tablespoon oat flour and 1½ teaspoons powdered sugar or xylitol to help thicken it.

GAME DAY VEGAN

DECADENT SNACKAGE THAT NOBODY WILL GUESS IS VEGAN

Buffalo Cauliflower Wings with Blue Cheese Dip

SERVES 4, WITH EXTRA DIP

PREP TIME: **10 minutes**
ACTIVE TIME: **20 minutes**   INACTIVE TIME: **15 minutes**

Olive oil spray
buffalo cauliflower
1 cup unsweetened nondairy milk (nut-free if necessary)
1 cup chickpea flour
2 tablespoons cornmeal (gluten-free if necessary)
½ teaspoon garlic powder
½ teaspoon smoked paprika
1 large or 2 small heads cauliflower (2 lb), broken into florets
1 cup hot sauce
2 tablespoons apple cider vinegar
1 tablespoon no-salt-added tomato paste
1 tablespoon maple syrup

blue cheese dip
½ cup plain coconut yogurt (or soy yogurt; unsweetened)
½ cup vegan mayonnaise
2 tablespoons white wine vinegar
½ teaspoon vegan Worcestershire sauce (gluten-free if necessary)
½ teaspoon salt
½ teaspoon garlic powder
¼ teaspoon onion powder
¼ teaspoon dried marjoram
¼ teaspoon dried oregano
Half a 14-ounce block extra firm tofu, drained and crumbled
Black pepper to taste

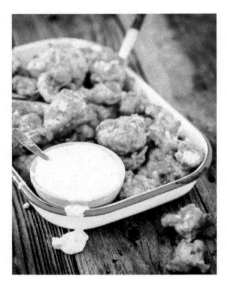

1. Preheat the oven to 450°F. Lightly spray a 9 × 13-inch baking dish with olive oil.

2. **To make the cauliflower** : Mix the milk, chickpea flour, cornmeal, garlic powder, and paprika in a large bowl. Dredge one cauliflower floret at a time in the mixture and place in the prepared baking dish. Bake for 20 minutes.

3. While the cauliflower is baking, mix together the hot sauce, apple cider vinegar, tomato paste, and maple syrup in a cup or small bowl.

4. Remove the cauliflower from the oven and use a spatula to loosen any florets sticking to the baking dish. Pour the hot sauce mixture over the cauliflower, toss to coat, and bake for 7 to 8 minutes more, until the hot sauce has thickened and caramelized.

5. While the cauliflower is baking the second time, **make the dip** : Mix the yogurt, mayonnaise, white wine vinegar, Worcestershire sauce, salt, garlic powder, onion powder, marjoram, and oregano in a medium bowl. Once combined, fold in the tofu. Taste and add pepper as needed.

6. Serve the cauliflower immediately with the dip. Leftovers will keep in airtight containers in the fridge for 2 to 3 days.

Jalapeño Popper Bites

MAKES 16 TO 18 POPPERS

PREP TIME: **15 minutes** (not including time to cook quinoa)
ACTIVE TIME: **25 minutes**

2 cups cooked quinoa
1 cup corn flour (certified gluten-free if necessary), plus more if needed
3 or 4 small jalapeños, seeded and chopped
2 tablespoons unsweetened nondairy milk (nut-free and/or soy-free if necessary; see Variations)
2 tablespoons lime juice
2 tablespoons vegan cream cheese or mayonnaise (soy-free if necessary)
3 tablespoons nutritional yeast
1 teaspoon ground cumin
½ teaspoon ground coriander
½ teaspoon smoked paprika
Salt and black pepper to taste
Sunflower or canola oil for frying
Salsa

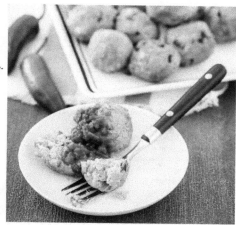

1. Combine the quinoa, corn flour, jalapeños, milk, lime juice, cream cheese or mayonnaise, nutritional yeast, cumin, coriander, and paprika in a large bowl and mix until fully combined. It should be moist and hold together when squeezed, but not wet like batter. If it's too wet, add corn flour by the tablespoon until you have the right consistency. Add salt and pepper.

2. Line a baking sheet with parchment paper or a silicone baking mat. Scoop about 2 tablespoons of the mixture into your hand and shape it into a ball. Place on the prepared baking sheet. Repeat with the remaining mixture.

3. Heat a large frying pan, preferably cast iron, over medium heat. Pour in enough oil to coat the bottom and heat for 2 to 3 minutes. It is important to give the oil enough time to heat. (The bites will fall apart if the oil is not hot enough.) Check to make sure it's hot enough by adding a pinch of the dough to the pan. If it sputters and sizzles, the oil is ready. Line a plate with paper towels.

4. Carefully place 5 or 6 bites in the pan and cook for 3 to 4 minutes, until golden and firm, flipping them every 30 seconds or so to cook on all sides. Use a slotted spoon to transfer them to the plate, placing more paper towels on top to absorb the excess oil. Repeat with the remaining bites, adding more oil to the pan as needed (allow the oil to heat each time you add more). Serve warm, with salsa for dipping. These are best eaten the same day but will keep in an airtight container in the fridge for 1 to 2 days.

VARIATIONS

▷ Make these poppers extra hot by replacing half or all of the milk with hot sauce.

▷ To bake the poppers instead of frying them, preheat the oven to 375ºF (190ºC), place the poppers on a baking sheet lined with parchment paper or a silicone baking mat, and bake for 30 minutes, flipping once halfway through.

Cheesy Spiced Popcorn

PREP TIME: **5 minutes**
ACTIVE TIME: **10 minutes**

3 tablespoons nutritional yeast
2 teaspoons chili powder
½ teaspoon garlic powder
A few pinches of cayenne pepper
2 tablespoons sunflower oil (or canola oil)
½ cup popcorn kernels
1 tablespoon vegan butter (soy-free if necessary, or coconut oil), melted
Salt to taste

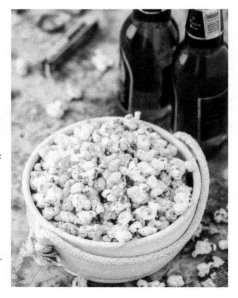

1. In a small cup or bowl, mix together the nutritional yeast, chili powder, garlic powder, and cayenne pepper. Set aside.

2. Combine the oil and 3 popcorn kernels in a large pot and heat over medium-high heat. Once the kernels pop, add the remaining kernels, cover the pot, shake it a couple of times, and return to the heat. Once the popping begins, continue to shake it every 3 to 5 seconds until the popping stops. Remove from the heat and uncover.

3. Pour the melted butter over the popcorn, cover the pot again, and shake to coat. Uncover the pot and add the nutritional yeast mix, cover again, and shake to coat. Uncover the pot and add salt. Serve immediately.

Chickpea-Avocado Taquitos

MAKES 8 TAQUITOS

PREP TIME: **5 minutes**
ACTIVE TIME: **25 minutes** INACTIVE TIME: **20 minutes**

1½ cups cooked chickpeas (or one 15-ounce can, rinsed and drained)
2 tablespoons liquid aminos (or gluten-free tamari; use coconut aminos to be soy-free)
1 avocado, pitted
2½ tablespoons lime juice
2 green onions, chopped (green and white parts)
1½ tablespoons plain vegan yogurt (or mayonnaise; soy-free if necessary), optional, to add creaminess
½ teaspoon ancho chile powder
½ teaspoon garlic powder
Salt and black pepper to taste
8 corn tortillas (see Tip)
Olive oil spray
Salsa or dip of your choice

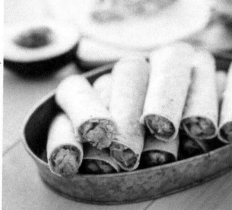

1. Preheat the oven to 350°F. Line a baking sheet with parchment paper or a silicone baking mat.

2. Heat a large frying pan, preferably cast iron, over medium heat. Add the chickpeas and liquid aminos and cook, stirring occasionally, until all the liquid has been absorbed. Remove from the heat and let cool for 2 to 3 minutes. Use a potato masher or pastry cutter to mash the chickpeas into small pieces.

3. Scoop the avocado flesh into a large bowl and mash until smooth but slightly chunky. Add the chickpeas, lime juice, green onions, yogurt (if using), ancho chile powder, garlic powder, salt, and pepper. Stir until combined.

4. Heat a frying pan over medium heat and heat the tortillas, one at a time, for 30 seconds on each side, until soft and pliable. Stack them on a plate and cover with aluminum foil while you cook the rest.

5. Lay out 1 tortilla and spread about 3 tablespoons of the avocado mixture down the center. Roll into a tube and place it seam side down on the prepared baking sheet. Repeat with the remaining tortillas and filling.

6. Spray the taquitos with olive oil and bake for 10 minutes. Flip the taquitos, spray them with olive oil again, and bake for another 10 minutes, or until crispy. Serve immediately with your choice of dip or salsa.

VARIATIONS

▶ You can make taquitos with a plethora of different fillings. Try Jackfruit Carnitas, 15-Minute Refried Beans with Pepperjack Cheese Sauce, Tempeh Sloppy Joes, or even Scrambled Tofu .

TIP

▶ Thin corn tortillas work best for these taquitos. Steer away from ones that say "handmade," as those are generally thicker and more likely to crack when you roll them up.

Pizzadillas

SERVES 2 TO 4

PREP TIME: **15 minutes** (not including time to make Pizza Sauce and Basic Cashew Cheese Sauce)
ACTIVE TIME: **20 minutes**

2 cups sliced fresh cremini mushrooms (or button mushrooms)
1 cup sliced green or red bell pepper
½ cup sliced red onion
2 cups loosely packed fresh spinach leaves
Salt and black pepper to taste
4 large flour tortillas (see Variation for making these gluten-free)
2 cups Pizza Sauce ; or store-bought vegan pizza or marinara sauce)
½ cup sliced pitted black olives
 Basic Cashew Cheese Sauce
Olive oil spray

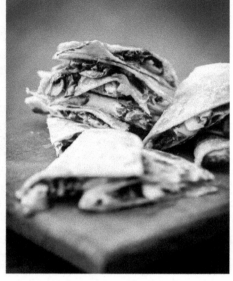

1. Heat a large frying pan over medium heat. Add the mushrooms, bell pepper, and onion and cook until the mushrooms are tender, 3 to 4 minutes. Add the spinach and cook until just beginning to wilt. Remove from the heat and add salt and pepper. Transfer to a bowl. Clean out the frying pan.

2. Lay out a tortilla. Spread tomato sauce on half. Top with a quarter of the veggies and a sprinkle of black olives. Drizzle about 3 tablespoons cheese sauce on top and fold over the other side of the tortilla. Repeat with the remaining ingredients.

3. Heat the frying pan over medium heat. Spray the pan with olive oil and add 2 quesadillas. Spray the tops of the quesadillas with olive oil. After 2 to 3 minutes, when the bottom is golden, flip the quesadillas and cook for 2 to 3 minutes more, until both sides are crispy and golden. Place them on a plate and cover with aluminum foil. Repeat with the remaining quesadillas. Slice and serve immediately, with a light drizzle of the cheese sauce over the top and the extra pizza sauce as a dip.

VARIATION

▶ To make these gluten-free, you'll need some large gluten-free tortillas. Since these tend to break when folded, the method will be a little different. Spread the pizza sauce, toppings, and cheese sauce over the entire tortilla, rather than just half. Top with another tortilla and cook as in step 3, repeating to make 2 total. Slice just as you would a normal pizza.

Cilantro Chile Almond Dip

MAKES 1¾ CUPS

PREP TIME: **10 minutes**
ACTIVE TIME: **10 minutes**
INACTIVE TIME: **2 hours**

1 cup raw almonds, soaked in warm water for at least 1 hour and drained, water reserved
1 cup reserved soaking water
1 cup roughly chopped fresh cilantro
¼ cup canned diced green chiles
¼ cup lime juice
2 tablespoons liquid aminos (or gluten-free tamari; use coconut aminos to be soy-free)
2 tablespoons chopped yellow onion
4 teaspoons nutritional yeast
2 teaspoons chopped garlic
1 teaspoon ground cumin
A few pinches of cayenne pepper
Salt and black pepper to taste

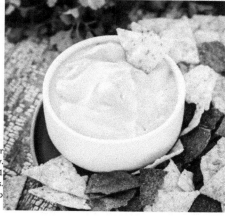

Combine all of the ingredients in a high-speed blender or food processor and blend until smooth and creamy. Transfer to an airtight container and refrigerate for 1 hour prior to serving. The dip should thicken as it chills. It will keep in an airtight container in the fridge for 2 to 3 days.

GET-TOGETHER VEGAN MEALS

SPECIAL MEALS FOR FANCIER GET-TOGETHERS

131

Avocado & Hearts of Palm Tea Sandwiches

MAKES 16 SANDWICHES

PREP TIME: **5 minutes**
ACTIVE TIME: **15 minutes**

2 avocados, pitted
2 teaspoons lemon juice
½ cup finely chopped hearts of palm
Salt and black pepper to taste
8 vegan bread slices (gluten-free if necessary; see Tip)
2 tablespoons chopped fresh parsley
1 cup very thinly sliced radishes

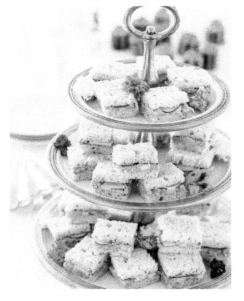

1. Scoop the avocado flesh into a medium bowl and mash until mostly smooth. Add the lemon juice, hearts of palm, salt, and pepper.

2. Spread the avocado mixture on 4 bread slices. Sprinkle with parsley and top with radish slices. Cover each with another piece of bread.

3. Use a bread knife to cut the crusts off each sandwich, then slice each sandwich into four triangles or squares. Serve immediately or refrigerate the sandwiches in an airtight container for up to 3 hours before serving.

TIP

▶ When using gluten-free bread, if you toast it lightly before using, it sometimes tastes better and doesn't dry out as much.

Roasted Red Pepper Hummus Cucumber Cups

MAKES 30 CUCUMBER CUPS

PREP TIME: **8 minutes**
ACTIVE TIME: **15 minutes**

roasted red pepper hummus

1½ cups cooked chickpeas (or one 15-ounce can, rinsed and drained)
½ cup chopped roasted red peppers
2 garlic cloves
3 tablespoons tahini (gluten-free if necessary)
3 tablespoons lemon juice
½ teaspoon smoked paprika
Pinch of cayenne pepper
Salt and black pepper to taste

cucumber cups

4 English cucumbers
Smoked paprika for dusting
Chives, sliced into 1-inch pieces

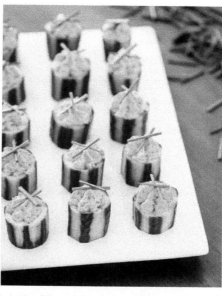

1. **To make the hummus** : Combine the ingredients in a food processor and process until smooth, pausing to scrape the sides as necessary. You may need to add water along the way to help smooth it out, but you want a thick hummus. Transfer the hummus to a pastry bag or a large resealable plastic bag with the corner cut out. Chill until ready to use.

2. Trim the ends of the cucumbers. Peel strips of skin from the sides of the cucumbers so you have a striped pattern. Alternatively, you can peel them completely, or not peel them at all. Slice the cucumbers into 1-inch sections. Use a melon baller or a teaspoon to hollow out the insides of the cucumbers, leaving a thick section at one end so that the "cup" has a bottom. Place all of the cups on a plate or platter.

3. Fill each cup with hummus, piling a little on top. Dust the tops with paprika and place 1 or 2 chive pieces on top. Refrigerate until you're ready to serve, up to 1 hour. Leftover hummus will keep refrigerated in an airtight container for 4 to 5 days.

Chickpea Caesar Pasta Salad

SERVES 6 TO 8

PREP TIME: **10 minutes** (not including time to make Pepita Parmesan)
ACTIVE TIME: **30 minutes**   INACTIVE TIME: **2 hours**

caesar dressing

¼ cup raw cashews, soaked in warm water for 1 hour and drained, water reserved
6 tablespoons reserved soaking water
¼ cup hemp seeds
3 tablespoons lemon juice
2 tablespoons olive oil
1 tablespoon vegan mayonnaise (soy-free if necessary), optional
1 tablespoon nutritional yeast
2 teaspoons vegan Worcestershire sauce (gluten-free and/or soy-free if necessary)
2 teaspoons Dijon mustard (gluten-free if necessary)
2 teaspoons drained capers
1 garlic clove
Salt and black pepper to taste

salad

12 ounces pasta shape of your choice (gluten-free if necessary)
3 cups cooked chickpeas (or two 15-ounce cans, rinsed and drained)
¼ cup liquid aminos (use coconut aminos to be soy-free)
2 cups halved cherry or grape tomatoes
1 large head romaine lettuce, chopped
2 avocados, pitted, peeled, and chopped
Pepita Parmesan

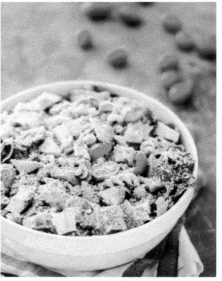

1. **To make the dressing** : Combine all of the ingredients in a food processor or blender and process until smooth. Set aside.

2. Bring a large pot of water to a boil and cook the pasta according to the package instructions until al dente. Drain, rinse the pasta with cold water, then drain again. Transfer the pasta to a large bowl.

3. Heat a large frying pan, preferably cast iron, over medium heat. Add the chickpeas and liquid aminos and cook, stirring occasionally, until all of the liquid has been absorbed, 4 to 5 minutes. Remove from the heat and add to the pasta.

4. Let the chickpeas cool for 5 to 10 minutes. Add the tomatoes, lettuce, and dressing and toss until combined. Gently fold in the avocado. Cover and refrigerate for 1 hour, or up to 3 hours, before serving. Serve topped with Pepita Parmesan (you can add it to the large bowl if people are serving themselves, or over individual servings if that's how you're serving it). This is best when eaten the day it's prepared but will keep in an airtight container in the fridge for about 1 day.

Sun-Dried Tomato & White Bean Bruschetta

SERVES 10 TO 12

PREP TIME: **10 minutes**
ACTIVE TIME: **15 minutes**

1 long vegan baguette (or other crusty bread; gluten-free if necessary)
1½ cups cooked cannellini beans (or one 15-ounce can, rinsed and drained)
¾ cups oil-packed sun-dried tomatoes, well drained and diced small
1 garlic clove, crushed
2 tablespoons fresh basil chiffonade
3 tablespoons white wine vinegar
Salt and black pepper to taste
½ cup toasted pine nuts (or other toasted nut or seed), optional
½ cup chopped green onions, optional

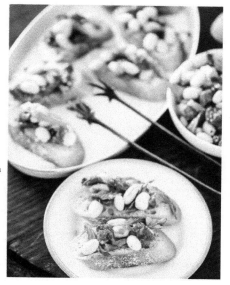

1. Preheat the oven to 350°F. Slice the bread into ½-inch slices and arrange them on a baking sheet. Bake for 7 to 10 minutes, until crispy and toasted. Set aside.

2. While the bread is toasting, mix together the beans, tomatoes, garlic, basil, vinegar, salt, and pepper.

3. Scoop some bean mixture onto each of the toasts and sprinkle the tops with pine nuts and green onions (if using). Serve immediately.

TIP

▶ You can prepare the bruschetta topping a few hours in advance and chill until ready to use.

▶ If you have leftover bean mixture, it makes a great filling for a wrap or sandwich.

135

Chickpea Croquettes with Dill Yogurt Sauce

SERVES 6 TO 8

PREP TIME: **20 minutes**
ACTIVE TIME: **50 minutes**

dill yogurt sauce

1 cup plain coconut yogurt (or soy yogurt; preferably unsweetened)
6 tablespoons vegan mayonnaise (soy-free if necessary)
¼ cup lemon juice
2 tablespoons freshly chopped dill (or 1 tbsp. dried dill)
2 teaspoons maple syrup (exclude if using sweetened yogurt)
1½ teaspoons garlic powder
1 teaspoon salt

croquettes

1 pound sweet potatoes or yams, peeled and roughly chopped
One 15-oz can chickpeas, brine reserved, chickpeas rinsed and drained
1 tablespoon reserved chickpea brine
4 green onions, finely chopped (green and white parts)
⅔ cup cornmeal (certified gluten-free if necessary)
1 garlic clove, crushed
1 teaspoon grated lemon zest
½ teaspoon paprika
Pinch of cayenne pepper
Salt and black pepper to taste
1 cup vegan panko bread crumbs (gluten-free if necessary)
Olive oil for frying

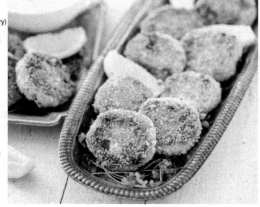

1. **To make the sauce** : Stir together the sauce ingredients in a medium bowl. Cover and refrigerate until ready to use.

2. **To make the croquettes** : Place the sweet potatoes in a pot and cover with water. Bring to a boil and cook for about 7 minutes, until tender. Drain well.

3. Place the chickpeas and 1 tablespoon brine in a large bowl and mash until broken into small pieces. Add the sweet potatoes and mash until mostly smooth. Add the green onions, cornmeal, garlic, lemon zest, paprika, cayenne pepper, salt, and pepper. Stir until combined.

4. Line a baking sheet with parchment paper or a silicone baking mat. Pour the bread crumbs into a shallow bowl. Scoop up an amount of the croquette mixture slightly larger than a golf ball, shape it into a patty, coat it in bread crumbs, and place it on the prepared baking sheet. Repeat with the remaining croquette mixture.

5. Line a plate with paper towels. Heat a large frying pan, preferably cast iron, over medium heat. Add enough olive oil to coat the bottom of the pan and let it heat until it shimmers. Add half of the croquettes and cook for 3 to 4 minutes on each side, until golden. Transfer to the plate to drain. Add more oil to the pan if needed (allow the oil to heat if you add more). Cook the remaining croquettes. Serve warm with the dill yogurt sauce. Leftovers will keep in airtight containers in the fridge for 2 to 3 days.

Champagne Cupcakes

MAKES 12 CUPCAKES

PREP TIME: **10 minutes**
ACTIVE TIME: **45 minutes** INACTIVE TIME: **40 minutes**

cupcakes

2 tablespoons nondairy milk (nut-free and/or soy-free if necessary)
1 tablespoon apple cider vinegar
1¾ cups unbleached all-purpose flour (or gluten-free flour blend, soy-free if necessary)
2 tablespoons arrowroot powder
1 cup coconut sugar
1 teaspoon baking powder
1 teaspoon baking soda
½ teaspoon salt
¼ teaspoon xanthan gum (exclude if using all-purpose flour or if your gluten-free blend includes it)
8 tablespoons vegan butter (soy-free if necessary), at room temperature
⅔ cup vegan Champagne
(or sparkling wine)
1 teaspoon vanilla extract

frosting

8 tablespoons vegan butter (soy-free if necessary)
3 cups powdered sugar (or xylitol)
2 tablespoons vegan Champagne (or sparkling wine)
½ teaspoon cream of tartar
½ teaspoon vanilla extract
Additional vegan decorations, optional

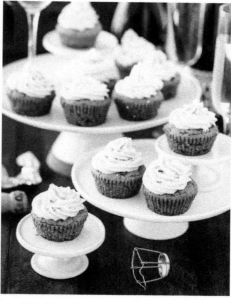

1. **To make the cupcakes** : Preheat the oven to 350°F. Line a 12-cup muffin tin with paper or silicone liners.

2. In a cup or small bowl, stir together the milk and vinegar. Set aside.

3. In a large bowl, whisk together the flour, arrowroot powder, coconut sugar, baking powder, baking soda, salt, and xanthan gum (if using).

4. In a medium bowl, use a hand mixer to cream together the butter and Champagne. Add the milk mixture and vanilla and mix until combined. Slowly add the wet ingredients to the dry ingredients and use the hand mixer to mix until combined.

137

5. Divide the mixture among the muffin cups and bake for 20 minutes, or until a toothpick inserted into the center comes out clean. Let the cupcakes cool in the muffin tin for 10 minutes before transferring them to a cooling rack to cool completely.

6. While the cupcakes are cooling, **make the frosting** : Use a hand mixer to mix all the frosting ingredients. Refrigerate for at least 15 minutes, or until ready to use.

7. Once the cupcakes are cool, transfer the frosting to a pastry bag fitted with a decorating tip or a large resealable plastic bag with the corner cut out, and use it to pipe frosting onto each cupcake. Alternatively, just use a butter knife or silicone spatula to spread frosting on each cupcake. You can add decorations if you like. Serve immediately or refrigerate until ready to serve. These cupcakes are best the day they're made but will keep in an airtight container in the fridge for 1 to 2 days.

VARIATION

▶ To make these alcohol-free, replace the Champagne with a vegan ginger ale or sparkling apple cider.

VEGAN BARBEQUES

VEGAN RECIPES BIG ENOUGH TO FEED A CROWD

Deviled Potato Salad

SERVES 4 TO 6

PREP TIME: **10 minutes**
ACTIVE TIME: **15 minutes**
INACTIVE TIME: **60 minutes**

1 pound baby Yukon gold potatoes (or baby Dutch Yellow Potatoes), quartered
¼ cup vegan mayonnaise (soy-free if necessary)
2 tablespoons vegan sweet pickle relish
1 tablespoon yellow mustard (gluten-free if necessary)
2 teaspoons apple cider vinegar
½ teaspoon onion powder
½ teaspoon garlic powder
½ teaspoon paprika, plus more for dusting
½ teaspoon black salt (kala namak; or regular salt)

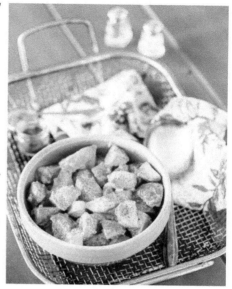

1. Place the potatoes in a pot and cover with water. Bring to a boil and cook the potatoes until easily pierced with a fork, 7 to 8 minutes. Drain, then rinse the potatoes with cold water until cool. Drain well.

2. Combine the mayonnaise, relish, mustard, vinegar, onion powder, garlic powder, paprika, and salt in a large bowl and stir until combined. Fold in the potatoes, letting them get mashed a little along the way. Lightly dust the top of the salad with more paprika and refrigerate for 1 hour before serving. Leftovers will keep in an airtight container in the fridge for 3 to 4 days.

Herbed Tofu Burgers

MAKES 6 BURGERS

PREP TIME: **10 minutes**
ACTIVE TIME: **45 minutes**
INACTIVE TIME: **30 minutes**

1 teaspoon olive oil
1 cup chopped yellow onion
2 garlic cloves, minced
One 14-ounce block extra firm tofu, pressed for about 30 minutes
2 tablespoons liquid aminos (or gluten-free tamari)
1 teaspoon v egan Worcestershire sauce (gluten-free if necessary)
½ teaspoon liquid smoke
½ teaspoon ground cumin
½ teaspoon dried thyme
½ teaspoon dried oregano
½ teaspoon dried basil
½ teaspoon dried parsley
¾ cup rolled oats (certified gluten-free if necessary)
½ cup vegan bread crumbs (gluten-free if necessary)
2 tablespoons sesame seeds
Salt and black pepper to taste
Olive oil spray
6 vegan burger buns (gluten-free if necessary)

Burger fixings (all are optional): lettuce, sliced tomato, sliced avocado, sliced red onion, pickles, 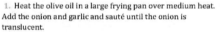 Pickled Red Cabbage & Onion Relish , ketchup, mustard, barbecue sauce, 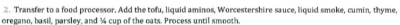 Basic Cashew Cheese Sauce or other vegan cheese

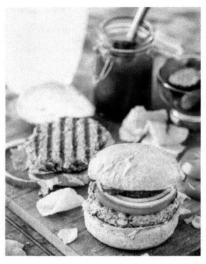

1. Heat the olive oil in a large frying pan over medium heat. Add the onion and garlic and sauté until the onion is translucent.

2. Transfer to a food processor. Add the tofu, liquid aminos, Worcestershire sauce, liquid smoke, cumin, thyme, oregano, basil, parsley, and ¼ cup of the oats. Process until smooth.

3. Transfer the mixture to a large bowl and add the remaining oats, the bread crumbs, and sesame seeds. Mix until combined. Add salt and pepper.

4. Line a baking sheet with parchment paper or a silicone baking mat. Divide the mixture into six equal parts. Using your hands or a greased biscuit cutter (sized to fit the buns), form the mixture into patties and place on the baking sheet.

5. Heat a large grill pan or frying pan, preferably cast iron, over medium heat. Generously spray the pan with olive oil. Place 2 or 3 patties in the pan (however many will fit without being crowded) and cook for 4 to 5 minutes on each side, a few minutes longer if your patties are more than ¾ inch thick, until firm, crisp, and browned on the outside. Place the burgers on buns. Repeat with the remaining patties, respraying the pan between batches.

6. Let everyone assemble their burger with their choice of fixings. Leftover burgers will keep in an airtight container in the fridge for up to 4 days.

Ranch-Seasoned Corn on the Cob

SERVES 4, WITH EXTRA SEASONING

PREP TIME: **5 minutes**
ACTIVE TIME: **25 minutes** INACTIVE TIME: **15 minutes**

ranch seasoning
2 tablespoons dried parsley
1 tablespoon dried minced onion
2 teaspoons onion powder
2 teaspoons garlic powder
1½ teaspoons dried dill
1½ teaspoons dried oregano
1 teaspoon celery seed
1 teaspoon salt
1 teaspoon coconut sugar
½ teaspoon paprika
¼ teaspoon black pepper

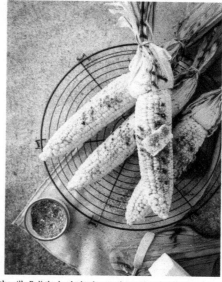

corn on the cob
At least 4 ears corn, in the husks (1 or more per person)
Vegan butter (soy-free if necessary)
Chopped fresh parsley, optional

1. **To make the ranch seasoning** : Combine all the ingredients in a food processor or spice grinder. Pulse a couple of times until it's a coarse powder. Transfer to a jar or airtight container.

2. **To make the corn on the cob** : Peel back the husks of the corn without detaching them. Remove and discard all the silk. Pull the husks back over the corn and place the ears in a large bowl or pot of cold water. Soak for 15 minutes.

3. Heat the grill to medium-high or heat a grill pan on the stove over medium heat. Place the corn on the grill and cook for 20 minutes, flipping once halfway through, or until the husks are slightly charred and the corn is tender.

4. If you want pretty grill marks on the corn, peel back the husks, place the corn directly on the grill, and cook for a couple of minutes on each side. Otherwise, just remove the corn from the grill.

5. Use a kitchen towel to pull back the husks. Tie them to form a handle. Spread butter over each ear and season generously with ranch seasoning. Sprinkle with chopped parsley (if desired) and serve immediately.

VARIATION

▶ You can also roast the corn. Remove the husks when you remove the silk and skip the soaking. Place each ear on a sheet of aluminum foil. Spread butter on the corn, then sprinkle generously with the ranch seasoning. Wrap the aluminum tightly around the corn. Roast at 450°F for 15 to 20 minutes, until the corn is tender.

TIP▶ You will have leftover spice blend, but don't worry—you can use this ranch seasoning just as you would any spice blend! Use it in the marinade for the Grilled Veggie Kebabs, sprinkle on the Perfect Roasted Potatoes before they go in the oven, or top your Quick & Easy Avocado Toast with it.

143

Creamy, Crunchy Coleslaw

SERVES 10 TO 12

PREP TIME: **15 minutes**
ACTIVE TIME: **20 minutes**
INACTIVE TIME: **35 minutes**

1 medium (1½- to 2-poundhead green cabbage,
quartered, cored, and shredded on a mandoline or
grater
2 medium carrots, peeled and grated
¾ cup vegan sugar
½ cup kosher salt
3 or 4 green onions, chopped (green and white parts)
¾ cup vegan mayonnaise (soy-free if necessary)
¼ cup apple cider vinegar
2 tablespoons maple syrup
2 teaspoons Dijon mustard (gluten-free if necessary)
1 teaspoon dried parsley
1 teaspoon celery seed
1 teaspoon black pepper
Salt to taste

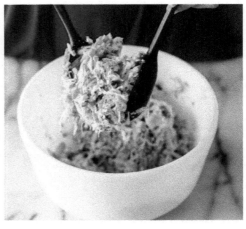

1. Combine the cabbage and carrots in a large bowl and toss with the sugar and kosher salt. Let rest for 5 minutes, then transfer to a colander and rinse thoroughly with cold water. (Not thoroughly rinsing the cabbage will result in overly salty slaw.) Rinse and dry the bowl. Run the cabbage and carrots through a salad spinner to remove the excess moisture, or spread out the mixture on a clean kitchen towel and pat dry with paper towels or another kitchen towel. Once dry, return the mixture to the bowl and add the green onions.

2. In a small bowl, mix together the mayonnaise, vinegar, maple syrup, mustard, parsley, celery seed, and pepper. Once thoroughly combined, add the dressing to the cabbage mixture and toss until evenly coated. Add salt if needed. Chill for at least 30 minutes before serving. Leftovers will keep in an airtight container in the fridge for 2 to 3 days.

Grilled Veggie Kebabs

MAKES 10 KEBABS

PREP TIME: **20 minutes**
ACTIVE TIME: **30 minutes**
INACTIVE TIME: **15 minutes**

¼ cup olive oil
3 tablespoons lemon juice
2 garlic cloves, minced
1 teaspoon dried basil
1 teaspoon dried parsley
½ teaspoon smoked paprika
10 medium cremini mushrooms (or button mushrooms), stemmed
10 cherry tomatoes
One 14- to 15-ounce can artichoke hearts, rinsed and drained
1 zucchini, sliced into ½-inch half circles
1 yellow squash, sliced into ½-inch half circles
1 red bell pepper, chopped into 1-inch squares
1 orange bell pepper, chopped into 1-inch squares
10 long wooden skewers

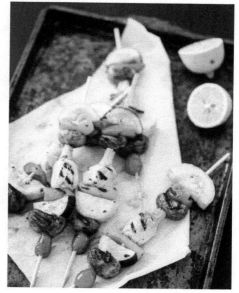

1. Combine the olive oil, lemon juice, garlic, basil, parsley, and paprika in a large shallow bowl or baking dish. Add the mushrooms, tomatoes, artichoke hearts, zucchini, squash, and bell peppers and toss to coat with the marinade. Marinate for about 15 minutes, tossing the veggies every few minutes or so. Soak the skewers in water while the veggies marinate.

2. Thread the veggies onto the skewers, making sure to get equal amounts of each veggie on each skewer.

3. Heat the grill to medium-high or heat a grill pan on the stove over medium-high heat. Cook the kebabs, brushing leftover marinade over them a couple of times, for 4 to 5 minutes per side, until tender and slightly charred. Serve immediately.

VARIATION

▷ Roasted Veggie Kebabs: Arrange the kebabs on a baking sheet lined with parchment paper or a silicone baking mat and roast them in a 450°F oven for 20 minutes, flipping once halfway through.

Rainbow Fruit Salad with Maple-Lime Dressing

SERVES 10 TO 12

PREP TIME: **25 minutes**
ACTIVE TIME: **5 minutes**
INACTIVE TIME: **60 minutes**

2 cups chopped strawberries
2 cups halved seedless green grapes
2 cups blueberries
1½ cups chopped fresh mango
1½ cups chopped fresh pineapple
One 11-ounce can mandarin oranges, rinsed,
drained, and cut in half
½ cup maple syrup
Grated zest and juice of 2 limes
2 tablespoons chopped fresh mint

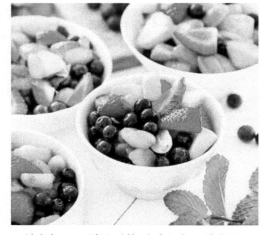

1. Combine the strawberries, grapes, blueberries, mango, pineapple, and mandarin oranges in a large bowl.

2. In a small bowl or cup, combine the maple syrup with the lime zest and juice. Add to the fruit, along with the mint, and toss until combined. Cover and refrigerate for 1 hour before serving. Leftovers will keep in an airtight container in the fridge for 1 to 2 days.

VEGAN HOLIDAYS

VEGAN DISHES THAT WILL START NEW HOLIDAY TRADITIONS

Cheesy Roasted Sweet Potatoes

SERVES 6 TO 8

PREP TIME: **5 minutes**
ACTIVE TIME: **5 minutes**
INACTIVE TIME: **35 minutes**

4 large sweet potatoes or yams (2 pounds), peeled and diced
Olive oil spray
4 to 6 tablespoons nutritional yeast
1 teaspoon garlic powder
1 teaspoon smoked paprika
Salt and black pepper to taste

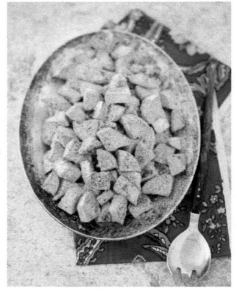

1. Preheat the oven to 425°F. Line two baking sheets with parchment paper or silicone baking mats.

2. Spread out the sweet potatoes on the sheets and spray with olive oil. Sprinkle the nutritional yeast, garlic powder, paprika, salt, and pepper over them and toss to coat.

3. Bake for 30 to 35 minutes, until easily pierced with a fork, tossing them once halfway through to ensure even cooking. Serve immediately. Refrigerate leftovers in an airtight container for 3 to 4 days.

Green Bean Casserole with Crispy Onion Topping

SERVES 6 TO 8

PREP TIME: **15 minutes** (not including time to make Cream of Mushroom Soup)
ACTIVE TIME: **25 minutes**
INACTIVE TIME: **25 minutes**

Olive oil spray
1 pound fresh green beans, trimmed

Cream of Mushroom Soup

1 tablespoon vegan butter (soy-free if necessary)
1 sweet onion, quartered and thinly sliced
¾ cup vegan panko bread crumbs (gluten-free if necessary)
½ teaspoon garlic powder
½ teaspoon salt
3 tablespoons nutritional yeast, optional

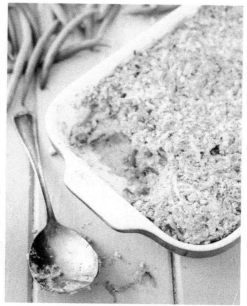

1. Preheat the oven to 400°F . Lightly spray a 9 × 13-inch baking dish with olive oil.

2. Place the green beans in a steamer basket over a pot of boiling water and cover. Steam for 5 minutes, then transfer to a large bowl. Pour the soup into the bowl and stir to combine. Set aside.

3. While the green beans are steaming, melt half of the butter in a large frying pan over medium heat. Add the onion and cook, stirring occasionally, until soft and golden, 5 to 7 minutes. Transfer the onions to a medium bowl. (Don't bother to clean the pan.) Melt the remaining butter in the frying pan and add the bread crumbs. Cook, stirring frequently, until the crumbs are crispy. Stir in the garlic powder and salt and remove from the heat. Add to the onions along with the nutritional yeast (if using). Stir to combine.

4. Pour the green bean mixture into the prepared baking dish. Spread the onion mixture over the top. Bake for 25 minutes, or until the topping is crispy and the casserole is bubbly. Serve immediately. Leftovers will keep in an airtight container in the fridge for 3 to 4 days.

TIP

▶ To prepare this in advance, bake the casserole without the topping for 25 minutes. Refrigerate until ready to serve. Prepare the onion topping, spread it on the top, and bake the casserole at 400°F for 15 to 20 minutes, until heated through.

Mashed Potatoes

SERVES 8 TO 10

PREP TIME: **10 minutes**
ACTIVE TIME: **10 minutes**

3 pounds Yukon gold potatoes, peeled and chopped into large chunks
½ cup unsweetened nondairy milk (nut-free and/or soy-free if necessary), plus more if needed
¼ cup olive oil
Salt and black pepper to taste

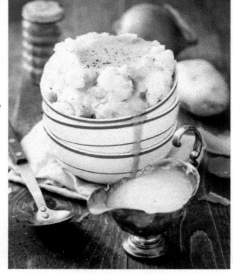

1. Place the potatoes in a pot and cover with water. Bring to a boil and cook until the potatoes are tender, 7 to 8 minutes. Drain the potatoes, then return them to the pot.

2. Add the milk and olive oil. Mash until it reaches the desired consistency. If the potatoes are still too dry, add milk by the tablespoon until it reaches the desired moisture level. Add salt and pepper. Leftovers will keep in the fridge in an airtight container for up to 4 days.

VARIATIONS

▶ Truffled Mashed Potatoes: Replace 3 tablespoons of the olive oil with truffle oil, and add ½ teaspoon of garlic powder.

▶ Reduced-Calorie Mashed Potatoes: Replace half of the potatoes with 1½ pounds cauliflower florets.

TIP

▶ To make the mashed potatoes extra smooth, process them in a food processor with the milk and olive oil.

Maple-Miso Tempeh Cutlets

SERVES 4

PREP TIME: **5 minutes**
ACTIVE TIME: **20 minutes**
INACTIVE TIME: **20 minutes**

Two 8-ounce packages tempeh
¼ cup low-sodium vegetable broth
¼ cup liquid aminos (or gluten-free tamari)
¼ cup maple syrup
2 teaspoons white soy miso (or chickpea miso)
1 teaspoon dried sage
1 teaspoon dried thyme
Salt and black pepper to taste

1. Chop each tempeh block in half horizontally, then chop each half diagonally so you have eight triangles.

2. Fill a large shallow saucepan with a couple of inches of water and fit with a steamer basket. Place the tempeh triangles in the steamer basket and cover with a lid. Bring to a boil, then reduce to a simmer. Steam the tempeh for 15 to 20 minutes, flipping the triangles once halfway through. Remove the steamer basket from the pan (keep the tempeh in the basket) and set aside.

3. Dump the water from the saucepan. Combine the vegetable broth, liquid aminos, maple syrup, miso, sage, and thyme in the pan and stir to mix. Add the tempeh triangles and bring to a boil. Once boiling, reduce the heat to a low simmer. Let the tempeh simmer in the sauce for 10 to 12 minutes, flipping them once halfway through, until the sauce is absorbed and starts to caramelize. Remove from the heat and add salt and pepper. Serve immediately. Leftovers will keep in an airtight container in the fridge for 4 to 5 days.

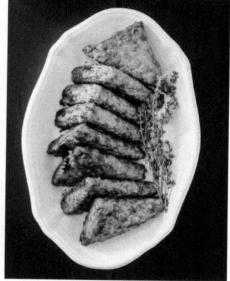

TIP

▶ For a killer Thanksgiving Leftovers Sandwich, slice one of the triangles widthwise so that you have two thinner triangles. Use those in the sandwich, along with some _Easy Tahini Gravy_, _Cheesy Roasted Sweet Potatoes_, and maybe some _Green Bean Casserole with Crispy Onion Topping_.

Easy Tahini Gravy

MAKES 3 CUPS

PREP TIME: **5 minutes**
ACTIVE TIME: **15 minutes**

1 tablespoon vegan butter (soy-free if necessary)
½ yellow onion, finely diced
1 teaspoon minced garlic
½ teaspoon dried thyme
½ teaspoon dried rosemary
2 tablespoons oat flour (certified gluten-free if necessary)
2½ cups low-sodium vegetable broth
2 tablespoons tahini (gluten-free if necessary)
2 tablespoons liquid aminos (or gluten-free tamari; use coconut aminos to be soy-free)
1 tablespoon nutritional yeast
Salt and black pepper to taste

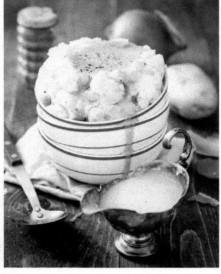

1. Melt the butter in a large shallow saucepan over medium heat. Add the onion and garlic and sauté until the onion is translucent, about 5 minutes. Add the thyme and rosemary and cook for a minute more. Add the flour and cook, stirring continuously, until the flour is completely incorporated.

2. Add the broth, tahini, and liquid aminos and stir until well combined. Cook, stirring frequently, until the gravy is thick and glossy, 5 to 7 minutes. Add the nutritional yeast and remove from the heat.

3. Use an immersion blender to blend the gravy until smooth. You can also transfer the gravy to a blender to blend until smooth. Add salt and pepper. Serve immediately. Leftovers will keep in an airtight container in the fridge for 2 to 3 days.

Marbled Pumpkin Cheesecake

SERVES 8 TO 10

PREP TIME: **15 minutes** (not including time to chill coconut cream)
ACTIVE TIME: **15 minutes**
INACTIVE TIME: **6 hours**

crust

1 cup Medjool dates, pitted
1½ cups pecan pieces
½ cup almond flour
½ teaspoon ground cinnamon
½ teaspoon ground ginger
½ teaspoon salt
2 tablespoons maple syrup
1 tablespoon coconut oil, melted
Vegan cooking spray (soy-free if necessary)

filling

1½ cups raw cashews, soaked in warm water for at least 4 hours and drained, water discarded (if you're using a high-speed blender, you can skip the soaking)
6 tablespoons chilled, hardened canned coconut cream (see Tip)
½ cup maple syrup
3 tablespoons lemon juice
1½ cups pureed pumpkin (not pumpkin pie filling)
1 teaspoon vanilla extract
1 teaspoon ground cinnamon
1 teaspoon ground ginger
½ teaspoon ground nutmeg
¼ teaspoon ground cloves
¼ teaspoon salt

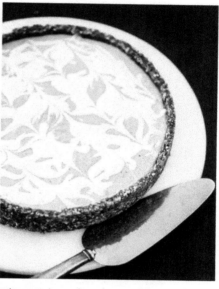

1. **To make the crust** : Place the dates in a food processor and process until they're in small pieces. Add the pecans and process until crumbly. Add the almond flour, cinnamon, ginger, salt, maple syrup, and coconut oil and process until incorporated and the mixture holds together when squeezed.

2. Line the bottom of a 9-inch springform pan with parchment paper and lightly spray the inside of the pan with cooking spray. Transfer the crust mixture to the pan and spread it evenly along the bottom and about 1 inch up the sides. Place the pan in the freezer.

3. **To make the filling** : In a blender, combine the cashews, coconut cream, maple syrup, and lemon juice. Blend until smooth, then transfer ¼ cup of the mixture to a small bowl and set aside. Add the pumpkin, vanilla, cinnamon, ginger, nutmeg, cloves, and salt to the processor. Blend until smooth. Pour on top of the crust and spread it evenly.

4. Drizzle the reserved cashew cream over the top. Carefully drag a toothpick or skewer through the coconut cream and pumpkin mixtures, making a marbleized pattern. Cover the pan, return to the freezer, and freeze for 2 hours. Transfer to the refrigerator until ready to serve. Remove the sides of the springform pan, slice, and serve. Leftovers will keep in the fridge for 3 to 4 days.

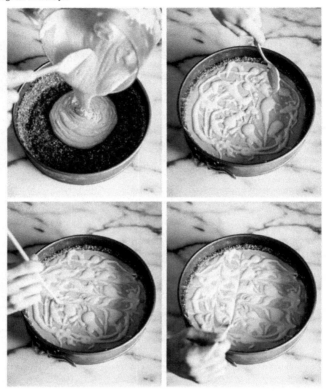

TIP ▷ Refrigerate a can of coconut cream or full-fat coconut milk overnight. The cream will harden and separate from the water. Use a can opener to open the can and lift off the lid. Carefully spoon out the solid coconut cream. Discard the water (or save it for later use). If you can find a 5.4-ounce can coconut cream, it will provide you with all the cream you need for this recipe.

Gingerbread Cookies

MAKES 24 COOKIES

PREP TIME: **10 minutes**
ACTIVE TIME: **20 minutes**   INACTIVE TIME: **45 minutes**

2 teaspoons flax meal
1 tablespoon warm water
¾ cup oat flour (certified gluten-free)
½ cup brown rice flour
¼ cup almond flour
1 tablespoon arrowroot powder
1 teaspoon baking soda
1 teaspoon ground ginger
½ teaspoon ground cinnamon
½ teaspoon salt
¼ teaspoon ground nutmeg
¼ teaspoon xanthan gum
⅓ cup coconut oil, melted
¼ cup blackstrap molasses (or regular molasses)
¼ cup coconut sugar (or brown sugar)
1 teaspoon grated fresh ginger
½ teaspoon vanilla extract

cinnamon sugar
3 tablespoons coconut sugar
1 tablespoon ground cinnamon

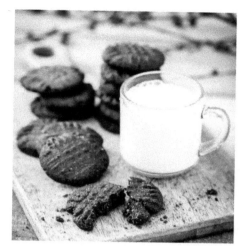

1. Mix the flax meal with the water in a medium bowl. Set aside and let rest for about 5 minutes.

2. Combine the oat flour, rice flour, almond flour, arrowroot, baking soda, ground ginger, cinnamon, salt, nutmeg, and xanthan gum in a large bowl and whisk until combined.

3. Add the coconut oil, molasses, sugar, grated ginger, and vanilla to the flax mixture. Mix until combined. Add the wet ingredients to the dry ingredients and stir until combined. Chill the dough in the fridge for at least 30 minutes.

4. Once you're ready to bake, preheat the oven to 350°F. Line two baking sheets with parchment paper or silicone baking mats. Remove the dough from the refrigerator.

5. **To make the cinnamon sugar** : Mix the sugar and cinnamon in a shallow bowl.

6. Scoop out a tablespoon of dough and roll it into a ball. Roll the ball in the cinnamon-sugar mixture, then place on the prepared baking sheet. Repeat with the remaining dough, spacing the balls about 2 inches apart. Use a fork to gently flatten each cookie and make a crisscross pattern on the top. Bake for 10 to 12 minutes, until the cookies are spread out and firm around the edges. Let the cookies cool on the pan for a couple of minutes before transferring them to a cooling rack. Cool completely before serving. (They will firm up more as they cool.) Store in an airtight container at room temperature for up 4 days.

VARIATION ▶ To make these cookies with gluten, replace the oat, brown rice, and almond flours with 1½ cups unbleached all-purpose flour and exclude the arrowroot powder and xanthan gum.

VEGANIZED FAMILY FAVORITES

CLASSIC FAMILY RECIPES (VEGANIZED) THAT EVEN GRANDMA WILL APPROVE OF!

IN THIS CHAPTER

Tempeh Sausage Minestrone

SERVES 8 TO 10

PREP TIME: **35 minutes**
ACTIVE TIME: **25 minutes** (not including time to make Quick Sausage Crumbles)
INACTIVE TIME: **20 minutes**

1 tablespoon olive oil
½ red onion, diced
2 medium carrots, peeled and sliced
2 celery stalks, sliced
½ fennel bulb, diced
2 cups sliced cremini mushrooms (or button mushrooms)
2 cups broccoli florets
2 small yellow squash, halved lengthwise and sliced
One 28-ounce can no-salt-added diced tomatoes
5 cups low-sodium vegetable broth
5 cups water
3 tablespoons liquid aminos (or gluten-free tamari; use coconut aminos to be soy-free)
2 teaspoons dried basil
2 teaspoons dried thyme
2 teaspoons dried oregano
½ teaspoon paprika
¼ teaspoon cayenne pepper
2 cups pasta (gluten-free if necessary)
1½ cups cooked great Northern beans (or one 15-ounce can, rinsed and drained)
1 cup frozen green peas
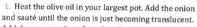
Quick Sausage Crumbles

2 cups packed chopped kale (or chard)
Salt and black pepper to taste

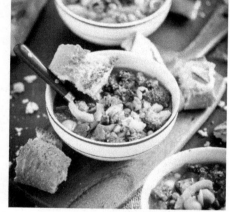

1. Heat the olive oil in your largest pot. Add the onion and sauté until the onion is just becoming translucent. Add the carrot, celery, fennel, and mushrooms and sauté for 2 to 3 minutes. Add the broccoli, squash, tomatoes and their liquid, broth, water, liquid aminos, basil, thyme, oregano, paprika, and cayenne pepper and bring to a boil. Reduce to a simmer and cook for about 10 minutes.

2. Add the pasta, beans, and peas and simmer until the pasta is al dente, about 10 minutes. Add the sausage crumbles, kale, salt, and pepper. Remove from the heat and serve immediately. Leftovers will keep in an airtight container in the fridge for 5 to 6 days, or frozen for up to 2 months.

157

Pot-obello Roast

SERVES 4 TO 6

PREP TIME: **20 minutes**
ACTIVE TIME: **35 minutes**   INACTIVE TIME: **20 minutes**

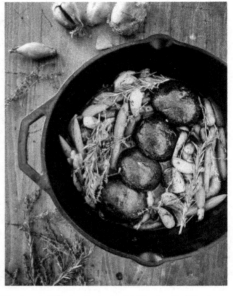

4 large portobello mushrooms
1 tablespoon olive oil
1 small red onion, quartered
6 shallots, trimmed and halved lengthwise
2 tablespoons brown rice flour (or other flour)
¼ cup vegan red wine
2 tablespoons liquid aminos (or gluten-free tamari; use coconut aminos to be soy-free)
1 tablespoon vegan Worcestershire sauce (gluten-free and/or soy-free if necessary)
1 teaspoon dried parsley
1 teaspoon salt
1 teaspoon black pepper
½ teaspoon paprika
3 cups vegan low-sodium "no-beef" flavored broth (or regular vegetable broth)
1 tablespoon nutritional yeast
1 pound small carrots, peeled (or baby carrots)
1 pound fingerling potatoes, halved lengthwise
8 ounces brussels sprouts, halved
4 thyme sprigs
2 rosemary sprigs

1. Remove the stems from the mushrooms and chop the stems into bite-size pieces. Set the stems and caps aside separately.

2. Preheat the oven to 400°F. Heat the oil in a large oven-safe pot or Dutch oven over medium heat. Add the onion and shallots and sauté for about 5 minutes, until softened. Add the flour and cook, stirring, until the flour is not visible, 1 to 2 minutes. Add the wine, liquid aminos, Worcestershire sauce, parsley, salt, pepper, and paprika and cook, stirring, for 2 to 3 minutes, until the mixture has thickened. Add the broth and stir in the nutritional yeast. Add the chopped mushroom stems, carrots, potatoes, and brussels sprouts and bring to a boil. Reduce the heat to a simmer and cook for about 5 minutes.

3. Remove from the heat. Arrange the portobello mushroom caps in the center of the pan, with vegetables surrounding and under them, and spoon sauce over the tops until well covered. Top with the thyme and rosemary sprigs. Cover the pot and place it in the oven. Roast for 15 minutes, then remove the lid and roast for another 5 minutes, uncovered. The mushrooms and vegetables should all be very tender. Remove from the oven.

4. You can serve straight from the pot, or arrange the portobello caps in the center of a platter surrounded by the vegetables and garnished with the herbs, and spoon the sauce over the top. Leftovers will keep in an airtight container in the fridge for 2 to 3 days.

Sweet Potato Casserole

SERVES 8

PREP TIME: **20 minutes**
ACTIVE TIME: **25 minutes**
INACTIVE TIME: **20 minutes**

casserole

4 pounds sweet potatoes or yams, peeled and roughly chopped
Vegan cooking spray (soy-free if necessary)
⅓ cup unsweetened nondairy milk (soy-free if necessary)
⅓ cup maple syrup
¼ cup coconut sugar (or brown sugar)
3 tablespoons vegan butter (soy-free if necessary; or coconut oil), melted
2 tablespoons lemon juice
1 tablespoon nutritional yeast, optional
1 teaspoon ground cinnamon
½ teaspoon ground ginger
½ teaspoon salt
¼ teaspoon ground nutmeg

topping

1½ cups chopped pecans
1 cup rolled oats (certified gluten-free if necessary)
1 cup vegan cornflakes (certified gluten-free if necessary)
⅓ cup oat flour (certified gluten-free if necessary)
¼ cup coconut sugar (or brown sugar)
1 teaspoon ground cinnamon
¼ teaspoon salt
4 tablespoons vegan butter (soy-free if necessary; or coconut oil), melted
1 tablespoon maple syrup

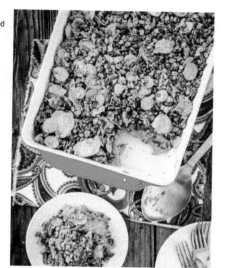

1. **To make the casserole** : Place the sweet potatoes in a large pot and cover with water. Bring to a boil and cook for 8 to 10 minutes, until tender. Remove from the heat and drain. Set aside.

2. Preheat the oven to 350°F. Lightly spray a 9 × 13-inch baking dish with cooking spray.

3. Transfer the sweet potatoes to a large bowl. Add the milk, maple syrup, sugar, butter, lemon juice, nutritional yeast (if using), cinnamon, ginger, salt, and nutmeg. Use a masher to mash and combine the mixture until mostly smooth. Transfer to the prepared baking dish.

4. **To make the topping** : Mix together the pecans, oats, cornflakes, oat flour, sugar, cinnamon, and salt. Pour the melted butter and maple syrup over the top and stir until combined. Spread the topping over the casserole.

5. Bake for 20 minutes, or until the topping is crispy and the casserole is heated through. Serve immediately. Leftovers will keep in an airtight container in the fridge for 3 to 4 days.

VARIATION ▶ For a richer flavor, instead of boiling the sweet potatoes, roast them whole for 1 hour at 400°F . Let them cool, then scoop the flesh from the skins.

Skillet Cornbread

SERVES 8

PREP TIME: **5 minutes**
ACTIVE TIME: **15 minutes**
INACTIVE TIME: **35 minutes**

Olive oil spray (or vegan cooking spray, soy-free if necessary)
1 cup unsweetened almond milk
1 teaspoon apple cider vinegar
¼ cup + 2 tablespoons warm water
2 tablespoons flax meal
1½ cups fine cornmeal (certified gluten-free if necessary)
1 cup oat flour (certified gluten-free if necessary)
¼ cup almond flour
1 tablespoon baking powder
½ teaspoon salt
½ teaspoon ground cumin
¼ teaspoon smoked paprika
¼ cup sunflower oil (or grapeseed oil)
¼ cup maple syrup

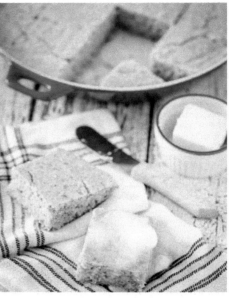

1. Preheat the oven to 400°F. Spray a 10-inch cast-iron skillet with olive oil.

2. In a 2-cup liquid measuring cup or a medium bowl, combine the milk with the vinegar. In a small cup or bowl, mix together the water and flax meal. Let both rest while you prepare the rest of the ingredients, or for 3 to 4 minutes

3. In a large bowl, whisk together the cornmeal, oat flour, almond flour, baking powder, salt, cumin, and paprika.

4. Once the flax meal mixture has thickened, add it to the milk. Add the sunflower oil and maple syrup. Stir until fully combined.

5. Add the wet ingredients to the dry ingredients and stir until just combined. Pour into the prepared skillet.

6. Bake for 20 to 25 minutes, until a toothpick inserted into the center comes out clean. Let rest for 5 to 10 minutes before serving. Leftovers will keep in an airtight container in the fridge for 2 to 3 days.

Grandma's Famous Date Nut Bread

MAKES 1 LOAF, 12 SLICES

PREP TIME: **15 minutes**
ACTIVE TIME: **15 minutes**
INACTIVE TIME: **75 minutes**

1 cup chopped pitted dates
¾ cup chopped walnuts
1½ teaspoons baking soda
½ teaspoon salt
⅛ teaspoon xanthan gum (exclude if using all-purpose flour or if your gluten-free blend includes it)
¾ cup boiling water
3 tablespoons vegan butter (soy-free if necessary)
Vegan cooking spray (soy-free if necessary)
½ cup unsweetened applesauce
1 tablespoon apple cider vinegar
1 teaspoon vanilla extract
1½ cups unbleached all-purpose flour (or gluten-free flour blend, soy-free if necessary)

1 cup coconut sugar (or brown sugar)

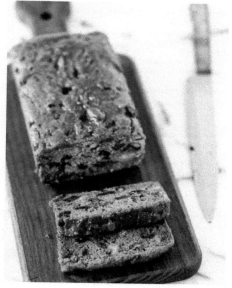

1. Combine the dates, walnuts, baking soda, salt, and xanthan gum (if using) in a medium bowl. Pour in the boiling water and stir in the butter. Let the mixture rest for 20 minutes.

2. Preheat the oven to 350°F. Spray a 9 × 5-inch loaf pan with cooking spray.

3. In a large bowl, stir together the applesauce, vinegar, and vanilla. Gradually stir in the flour and sugar. It will be lumpy, and that's okay; just incorporate everything as thoroughly as you can. Add the date mixture and stir until combined. Pour into the prepared loaf pan.

4. Bake for 50 to 55 minutes, until a toothpick inserted in the center comes out clean. Let cool in the pan for 15 minutes before transferring to a cooling rack. Cool for at least 4 hours before slicing. Leftovers can be stored in an airtight container at room temperature for 3 to 4 days.

Peanut Butter Pie

MAKES 8 SLICES

PREP TIME: **10 minutes** (not including time to chill coconut cream)
ACTIVE TIME: **25 minutes**   INACTIVE TIME: **2 hours + 10 minutes**

Vegan cooking spray (soy-free if necessary)
crust
1 cup oat flour (certified gluten-free if necessary)
½ cup almond flour
¼ cup coconut sugar (or brown sugar)
1 tablespoon arrowroot powder
1 teaspoon ground cinnamon
½ teaspoon vanilla powder, optional
½ teaspoon baking soda
½ teaspoon salt
6 tablespoons very cold vegan butter (soy-free if necessary)
1 teaspoon apple cider vinegar
filling
1 cup unsalted, unsweetened, smooth natural peanut butter
One 12-ounce vacuum-packed block extra firm silken tofu
5 tablespoons chilled, hardened canned coconut cream (see Tip)
½ cup coconut sugar (or brown sugar)
2 tablespoons tapioca powder
1 teaspoon vanilla extract
½ teaspoon salt
peanut butter crumble
¼ cup unsalted, unsweetened, smooth natural peanut butter
¼ cup oat flour (certified gluten-free if necessary)
¼ cup powdered sugar (or xylitol)

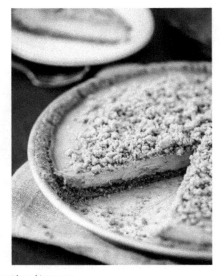

1. Preheat the oven to 375°F . Lightly spray a 9-inch pie pan with cooking spray.

2. **To make the crust** : In a large bowl, whisk together the oat flour, almond flour, sugar, arrowroot, cinnamon, vanilla powder (if using), baking soda, and salt. Cut in the butter and vinegar until it has the texture of wet sand and no pieces are larger than your pinkie fingernail.

3. Pour the mixture into the pie pan and use your hands to evenly distribute and spread the crust along the bottom and up the sides. Bake for 10 minutes. Remove from the oven and let cool completely before adding the filling.

4. **To make the filling** : In a food processor, combine the peanut butter, tofu, coconut cream, sugar, tapioca powder, vanilla, and salt. Process until smooth. Pour into the prepared crust. Refrigerate until ready to use.

5. **To make the crumble** : In a small bowl, combine the ingredients and stir with a fork until crumbly. Sprinkle the crumbles over the top of the pie. Chill for at least 2 hours, or until ready to serve. Leftovers will keep in an airtight container in the fridge for 1 to 2 days.

TIP▸ Refrigerate a can of coconut cream or full-fat coconut milk overnight. The cream will harden and separate from the water. Use a can opener to open the can and lift off the lid. Carefully spoon out the solid coconut cream. Discard the water (or save it for later use). If you can find a 5.4-ounce can coconut cream, it will provide you with all the cream you need for this recipe.

ROMANTIC VEGAN

ROMANTIC VEGAN MEALS THAT WILL REALLY SET THE MOOD

163

Silky Cheese Fondue

SERVES 6 TO 8

PREP TIME: **20 minutes**
ACTIVE TIME: **35 minutes**
INACTIVE TIME: **60 minutes**

8 ounces fingerling potatoes (or baby Dutch Yellow Potatoes)
1½ cups raw cashews, soaked in warm water for at least 1 hour and drained, water reserved
¾ cup reserved soaking water
3 tablespoons nutritional yeast
2 tablespoons sauerkraut
2 tablespoons refined coconut oil
½ teaspoon onion powder
½ teaspoon garlic powder
1 cup vegan dry white wine
¼ cup water
3 tablespoons tapioca powder
Salt, optional

suggested dippers

Cubed vegan bread (gluten-free if necessary)
Cherry tomatoes
Chopped roasted or steamed veggies, such as carrots, mushrooms, asparagus, broccoli, cauliflower, or even potatoes or sweet potatoes
Fresh fruit, such as apple or pear slices or grapes

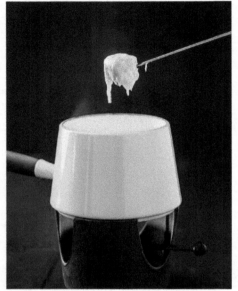

1. Place the fingerling potatoes in a medium pot and cover with water. Boil until tender, 7 to 8 minutes. Remove from the heat and drain. Transfer the potatoes to a blender along with the cashews, reserved soaking water, nutritional yeast, sauerkraut, coconut oil, onion powder, and garlic powder. Blend until smooth, then transfer to the medium pot. Cook over medium heat, stirring occasionally, until heated through, about 5 minutes. Reduce the heat to medium-low. Add the wine and cook for another 5 minutes.

2. In a cup or small bowl, whisk together the water and tapioca powder. Add to the pot and cook, stirring constantly, until the fondue is thick and glossy. Add salt, if desired. Remove from the heat and transfer to a double boiler or a fondue pot over a tea light candle. Serve immediately with the dippers of your choice. Leftovers can be refrigerated in an airtight container for 1 to 2 days.

Avocado, Pomegranate & Pine Nut Salad

SERVES 2 TO 4

PREP TIME: **15 minutes**
ACTIVE TIME: **5 minutes**

citrus-chili vinaigrette

¼ cup orange juice
2 tablespoons Champagne vinegar (or white wine vinegar)
1 tablespoon maple syrup
2 teaspoons olive oil
½ teaspoon chili powder

salad

3 cups packed mixed baby greens
1 avocado, pitted, peeled, and chopped
1 cup diced strawberries
½ cup pomegranate seeds
¼ cup toasted pine nuts

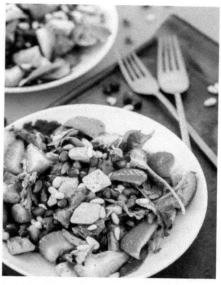

1. In a cup or small bowl, stir together the vinaigrette ingredients.

2. In a large bowl, toss together the greens, avocado, strawberries, pomegranate seeds, and pine nuts. Add the dressing and toss until evenly coated. Divide between two bowls and serve immediately.

VARIATION

▶ To liven up the salad a bit or turn it into more of a main course, add some cooked chickpeas, Quick Bacon Crumbles, or Chile-Roasted Tofu . A little sprinkling of Pepita Parmesan never hurt anybody either.

165

Deconstructed Sushi Bowl

SERVES 2 TO 4

PREP TIME: **45 minutes** (not including time to cook rice and make Lemongrass Tofu or Chile-Roasted Tofu)
ACTIVE TIME: **15 minutes**

sushi bowl

1 large or 2 small watermelon radishes, thinly sliced (see Tip)
Salt to taste
3 cups cooked white sushi rice (or short-grain black rice)
Lemongrass Tofu or Chile-Roasted Tofu

3 small carrots, peeled and julienned
1 cucumber or ½ English cucumber, thinly sliced
1 avocado, pitted, peeled, and thinly sliced
1 or 2 nori sheets
¼ cup sliced green onions (green and white parts)
Pickled ginger
Black and/or white sesame seeds

dressing

3 tablespoons gluten-free tamari
2 tablespoons brown rice vinegar
1 tablespoon mirin

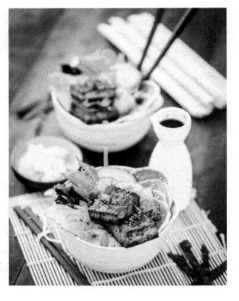

1. Ten minutes before serving, lay out the radish slices on a few paper towels. Sprinkle with salt and let them drain until ready to serve.

2. Divide the rice between two bowls. Top with pieces of tofu, carrots, cucumbers, radishes, and avocado.

3. Slice the nori sheet in half lengthwise. Slice each half widthwise into thin strips. Top each bowl with the nori strips, green onions, a bit of pickled ginger, and sesame seeds.

4. Combine the tamari, vinegar, and mirin in a small cup or bowl. Drizzle over each bowl. Serve immediately. Leftovers will keep in an airtight container in the fridge for 2 to 3 days.

TIP

▶ If you can't find watermelon radishes, you can use 5 or 6 regular radishes, very thinly sliced.

Sun-Dried Tomato Linguine

SERVES 4 (MAKES 6 CUPS/1.4 L SAUCE)

PREP TIME: **15 minutes** (not including time to make Pepita Parmesan)
ACTIVE TIME: **30 minutes**
INACTIVE TIME: **10 minutes**

sun-dried tomato marinara sauce
4 ounces sun-dried tomatoes, chopped
2 cups warm water
1 teaspoon olive oil
½ medium yellow onion, diced
2 garlic cloves, peeled
2 cups halved cherry tomatoes
½ cup chopped fresh basil
One 15-ounce can no-salt-added tomato sauce
One 6-ounce can no-salt-added tomato paste
2 teaspoons maple syrup
Black pepper to taste

1 pound linguine (gluten-free if necessary)
Pepita Parmesan, optional

½ cup sliced pitted green olives
2 tablespoons capers, rinsed and drained
Chopped fresh parsley or basil, optional

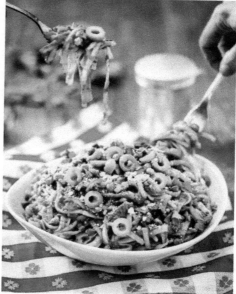

1. Place the sun-dried tomatoes in a bowl and cover with the water. Let them soak for 10 minutes, or until rehydrated and tender. Drain, and reserve the soaking water.

2. Heat the olive oil in a large saucepan over medium heat. Add the onion and garlic and sauté until the onion is translucent. Add the sun-dried tomatoes and cherry tomatoes and cook, stirring occasionally, for about 8 minutes, until tender. Stir in the basil, tomato sauce, tomato paste, 1½ cups of the reserved soaking water, and the maple syrup. Stir until combined.

3. Use an immersion blender to blend the mixture until smooth (or mostly smooth), or transfer to a blender and blend until smooth. Simmer for 10 minutes more, stirring occasionally. If the sauce is sputtering too much, reduce the heat to medium-low. Add pepper.

4. While the sauce is cooking, bring a large pot of water to a boil. Add the linguine and cook according to the package instructions until al dente. Drain.

5. You can either add the pasta to the sauce or serve the pasta with the sauce spooned over it. Either way, garnish with a sprinkle of Pepita Parmesan (if using), olives, capers, and parsley (if using). Serve immediately. Leftovers will keep in an airtight container in the fridge for 3 to 4 days.

Scallops with Creamy Mushroom-Leek Sauce

SERVES 2

PREP TIME: **10 minutes**
ACTIVE TIME: **30 minutes**

4 large, thick-stemmed king trumpet mushrooms (see Tip)
2 tablespoons vegan butter (soy-free if necessary)
Salt and black pepper to taste
1 large leek, thinly sliced (white and light green parts) and
thoroughly rinsed
1 garlic clove, minced
1 tablespoon fresh thyme leaves (or 1 teaspoon dried thyme)
1 tablespoon brown rice flour (or other gluten-free flour)
½ cup vegan white wine
½ cup unsweetened nondairy milk (nut-free and/or soy-free if
necessary)
Salt and black pepper to taste

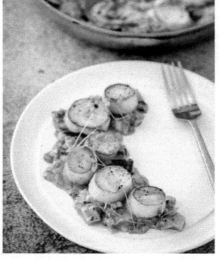

1. Rinse the mushrooms and pat them dry. Trim the caps off the mushrooms, then dice the caps into small pieces and set aside. Slice the stems into ¾- to 1-inch "scallops."

2. Melt 1 tablespoon of the butter in a large frying pan over medium heat. Season the scallops with salt and pepper and place them in the pan, flat side down. Cook for 2 to 3 minutes, until slightly crispy and golden on the bottom, then flip them. Cook for 2 to 3 minutes on the other side, until crispy and golden, then transfer them to a plate.

3. Melt the remaining butter in the pan. Add the leeks and the chopped mushroom caps and cook for about 3 minutes, until the leeks are soft. Add the garlic and thyme and cook for another minute. Add the flour and cook, stirring constantly, until the flour is fully incorporated. Add the wine and cook, stirring occasionally, until the liquid has reduced by half, about 3 minutes. Add the milk and cook, stirring frequently, until thick and creamy, about 4 minutes. Add salt and pepper.

4. Return the scallops to the pan and spoon the sauce over them. Heat them for a minute or two before serving. These are best eaten as soon as they are prepared.

TIP

▶ King trumpet mushrooms can be found in natural food stores such as Whole Foods and some Asian markets. You want to choose the longest, thickest-stemmed mushrooms you can find.

Mini Salted Chocolate Caramel Pretzel Tarts

SERVES 2

PREP TIME: **10 minutes**
ACTIVE TIME: **20 minutes** INACTIVE TIME: **2 hours + 25 minutes**

Vegan cooking spray (soy-free if necessary)

pretzel crust
1 heaping cup broken pretzels (gluten-free if necessary)
2 tablespoons coconut sugar (or brown sugar)
⅓ cup oat flour (certified gluten-free if necessary)
3½ tablespoons vegan butter (soy-free if necessary)

caramel layer
⅓ cup chopped pitted Medjool dates
⅓ cup full-fat coconut milk
1 tablespoon maple syrup
½ teaspoon vanilla extract
¼ teaspoon salt

chocolate ganache
2 heaping tablespoons vegan dark chocolate chips (or chopped vegan chocolate)
¼ cup full-fat coconut milk
1 teaspoon coconut oil, melted
Flaked sea salt, optional

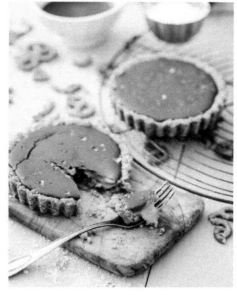

1. Preheat the oven to 350°F. Lightly spray two 4½-inch tart pans with cooking spray.

2. **To make the crust** : Combine the pretzels, sugar, and oat flour in a food processor and process into a coarse flour. Transfer to a large bowl and cut in the butter until it's a crumbly dough that holds together when squeezed.

3. Divide the dough between the two tart pans and press into the bottom and up the sides. Bake for about 12 minutes, until dark golden brown. Cool completely in the pans on a cooling rack.

4. **To make the caramel** : Combine the ingredients in a food processor. Process until smooth. Divide the mixture between the two crusts and refrigerate for 30 minutes.

5. **To make the ganache** : Place the chocolate in a heatproof bowl. Bring the coconut milk to a boil over medium heat, then immediately remove from the heat and pour over the chocolate. Let it rest for a few minutes before gently stirring until smooth. Stir in the coconut oil. Pour the ganache over the tarts and spread it out evenly. Sprinkle the tops with flaked sea salt, if desired.

6. Refrigerate the tarts until the chocolate is firm, at least 1 to 2 hours. Keep chilled until ready to serve. Leftovers will keep in airtight containers in the fridge for 2 to 3 days.

VEGAN HOMEMADE EDIBLE GIFTS

HOMEMADE EDIBLE GIFTS TO SHOW YOUR FAMILY YOUR APPRECIATION

IN THIS CHAPTER

Rescue Puppy Chow

Caramel Cashew Granola

Wild Rice, Mushroom & Lentil Soup in a Jar

Make-Your-Own Cornbread in a Jar

Apricot Pistachio Chocolate Bark

Spiced Nuts

Rescue Puppy Chow

MAKES 9 CUPS

PREP TIME: **5 minutes**
ACTIVE TIME: **15 minutes**
INACTIVE TIME: **30 minutes**

8 cups vegan waffle square cereal (such as Chex, using a gluten-free variety if necessary)
1 cup vegan chocolate chips (or chunks)
½ cup unsalted, unsweetened, smooth natural peanut butter
2 tablespoons vegan butter (soy-free if necessary)
1 teaspoon vanilla extract
¼ teaspoon salt
1 cup powdered sugar (or xylitol)

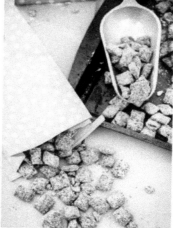

1. Pour the cereal into a very large bowl. Set aside.

2. Melt the chocolate in a double boiler or a heatproof bowl on top of a pot of boiling water, stirring frequently, until smooth. Stir in the peanut butter, butter, vanilla, and salt. Stir until combined and completely melted and smooth.

3. Pour the chocolate mixture over the cereal. Stir until combined. Add the powdered sugar and toss until fully coated.

4. Spread out the mixture on a baking sheet to cool completely. Divide among gift bags or jars, or place in an airtight container. You can refrigerate it, or store it at room temperature, where it will keep for 5 to 7 days.

VARIATION

▷ For the peanut butter fanatics in the family, try switching out the waffle cereal with puffed peanut butter cereal (such as Barbara's Peanut Butter Puffins).

Caramel Cashew Granola

MAKES 14 CUPS

PREP TIME: **10 minutes**
ACTIVE TIME: **20 minutes**
INACTIVE TIME: **40 minutes**

10 Medjool dates, pitted
½ cup nondairy milk (soy-free if necessary)
2 tablespoons maple syrup
2 tablespoons melted coconut oil
2 teaspoons vanilla extract
½ teaspoon salt
2½ cups rolled oats (certified gluten-free if necessary)
2½ cups puffed rice (or puffed millet)
1 cup buckwheat groats (kasha)
1½ cups chopped cashews (raw or toasted)
½ cup hemp seeds
2 tablespoons flax meal
2 teaspoons ground cinnamon
3 tablespoons coconut sugar (or brown sugar)

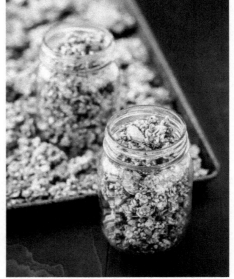

1. Position two racks in the oven near the center. Preheat the oven to 275°F. Line two baking sheets with parchment paper or silicone baking mats.

2. Combine the dates, milk, maple syrup, coconut oil, vanilla, and salt in a food processor or high-speed blender and process until smooth, pausing to scrape the sides as necessary. Set aside.

3. In a large bowl, stir together the oats, puffed rice, buckwheat groats, cashews, hemp seeds, flax meal, and cinnamon. Add the date mixture and stir until combined. Sprinkle the sugar over the granola and gently stir it in.

4. Spread out the granola over the two baking sheets and bake for 20 minutes. Switch the sheets, placing the bottom sheet on the upper rack and the top sheet on the lower rack, and bake for another 20 minutes, until crisp and golden. Let cool completely before crumbling and transferring to gift jars or an airtight container. The granola will keep at room temperature for about 2 weeks.

VARIATION
▶ For a sweeter granola, increase the sugar to ⅓ cup.

Wild Rice, Mushroom & Lentil Soup in a Jar

MAKES TWO 1-QUART JARS

PREP TIME: **5 minutes**
ACTIVE TIME: **10 minutes**

½ cup dried onion flakes
¼ cup nutritional yeast
1 tablespoon dried thyme
1 tablespoon dried parsley
1 tablespoon dried rosemary
2 teaspoons garlic powder
1 teaspoon paprika
1 teaspoon salt
½ teaspoon black pepper
1½ cups green or brown lentils
4 bay leaves
1½ cups wild rice
1 cup yellow split peas
2 cups roughly chopped dried shiitake mushrooms (or porcini mushrooms, or a mix)

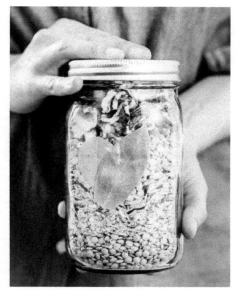

1. Combine the onion flakes, nutritional yeast, thyme, parsley, rosemary, garlic powder, paprika, salt, and pepper in a cup or small bowl and stir until well incorporated.

2. Pour ¾ cup of the lentils into each jar. Divide the spice mixture between the two jars. Place two bay leaves in each jar, pressed up against the side, with the bottom tips secured in the lentils and spices. Holding the leaves in place, pour ¾ cup of the rice into each jar. Once the rice is holding the leaves in place, you can let go of them.

3. Pour ½ cup of the split peas into each jar. Top each jar with 1 cup of the dried mushrooms. Tightly secure the lid on each jar. Attach a card with the following instructions to the jar:

- Combine the contents of the jar with 1 quart low-sodium vegetable broth in a large pot. Bring to a boil, then reduce to a simmer, cover, and cook for 25 minutes. Add 2 cups water, bring to a boil again, and reduce to a simmer. Cook uncovered for 20 minutes more, or until the lentils and split peas are tender. Add another 2 cups broth or water and simmer until heated through, about 5 minutes. Remove from the heat and add salt and pepper to taste. For an extra punch of flavor when serving, add a squeeze of lemon juice or a sprinkling of chopped fresh parsley. Enjoy! (Serves 6)

TIP

▶ To make the gift even more special, deliver it with a couple of large mugs and soup spoons.

173

Make-Your-Own Cornbread in a Jar

MAKES TWO 1-QUART JARS

PREP TIME: **5 minutes**
ACTIVE TIME: **5 minutes**

3 cups fine cornmeal (certified gluten-free if necessary)
3 cups unbleached all-purpose flour (or gluten-free flour blend, soy-free if necessary)
¼ cup coconut sugar (or brown sugar)
¼ cup flax meal
2 tablespoons baking powder
1 teaspoon baking soda
1 teaspoon salt

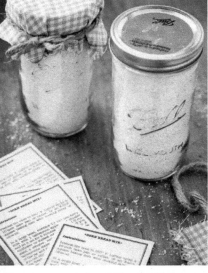

Whisk all the ingredients together in a large bowl. Divide evenly between the two jars. Tightly secure the lid on each jar. Attach a card with the following instructions to the jar:

- Preheat the oven to 350°F (180ºC). Lightly coat a 10-inch cake pan or skillet or an 8 × 8-inch baking dish with cooking spray or olive oil.
- In a large bowl, combine 1¼ cups nondairy milk with 1 tablespoon apple cider vinegar and let it sit for 5 minutes. Whisk in ⅓ cup sunflower oil or melted coconut oil. If you want a sweeter, moister cornbread, add 2 tablespoons maple syrup. Add the contents of the jar and stir until smooth. If you like, you can stir in 1 cup fresh corn kernels OR 1 cup fresh blueberries OR ¼ cup canned diced green chiles OR 2 tablespoons diced jalapeños.
- Pour the batter into the prepared pan and bake for 20 to 25 minutes, until a toothpick inserted into the center comes out clean. Let it rest for 10 minutes before serving. Enjoy! (Serves 8 to 10)

Apricot Pistachio Chocolate Bark

SERVES 10 TO 12

PREP TIME: **10 minutes**
ACTIVE TIME: **15 minutes**
INACTIVE TIME: **60 minutes**

2½ cups vegan dark chocolate chunks (or chips; soy-free if necessary)
2 teaspoons coconut oil
⅓ cup roughly chopped pistachios
Heaping ½ cup chopped dried apricots
Flaked sea salt

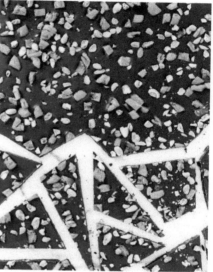

1. Line a baking sheet with parchment paper or a silicone baking mat. If possible, use binder clips to clip the edges of the paper to the rim of the sheet. This will hold it in place when you're spreading the chocolate.

2. Melt the chocolate with the coconut oil in a double boiler or a heatproof bowl on top of a pot of boiling water, stirring frequently, until smooth.

3. Pour the chocolate onto the prepared baking sheet and use a silicone spatula to spread it until it's about ¼ inch (6 mm) thick. Sprinkle the top with the pistachios and apricots, then with salt. Refrigerate for 1 hour, or until completely set.

4. Break the bark into pieces and place the pieces in cellophane bags tied closed with string or in a cute box. Store in a cool, dry place.

VARIATIONS

▶ You can, of course, use different dried fruits and/or nuts in this bark. Just use equal quantities as listed and you'll be golden.

▶ For a nut-free option, use shelled sunflower seeds or pepitas (pumpkin seeds).

TIP

▶ To really make this bark stand out, use high-quality, high-cacao-content chocolate.

Spiced Nuts

MAKES ABOUT 5½ CUPS

PREP TIME: **10 minutes**
ACTIVE TIME: **15 minutes**
INACTIVE TIME: **30 minutes**

1½ cups cashews
1½ cups almonds
1½ cups pecans
1 cup peanuts
¼ cup coconut sugar (or brown sugar)
3 tablespoons coconut oil, melted
3 tablespoons maple syrup
1 tablespoon lemon juice
1 tablespoon chili powder
2 teaspoons ground cumin
1 teaspoon ground cinnamon
Pinch of cayenne pepper
Flaky sea salt or kosher salt to taste

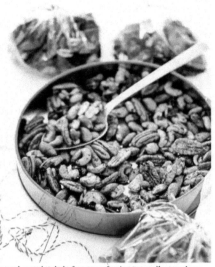

1. Preheat the oven to 350°F. Line a baking sheet with parchment paper or a silicone baking mat.

2. Combine the cashews, almonds, pecans, and peanuts in a large bowl. In a small bowl, stir together the coconut sugar, coconut oil, maple syrup, lemon juice, chili powder, cumin, cinnamon, and cayenne pepper. Pour over the nuts and toss until combined. Spread out the nuts on the baking sheet and sprinkle with salt.

3. Bake for 18 to 20 minutes, stirring twice with a
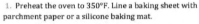
spatula, until the nuts are golden brown and glazed. Let them cool completely before transferring to small paper bags or jars or a large airtight container. The nuts will keep at room temperature for 4 to 5 days.

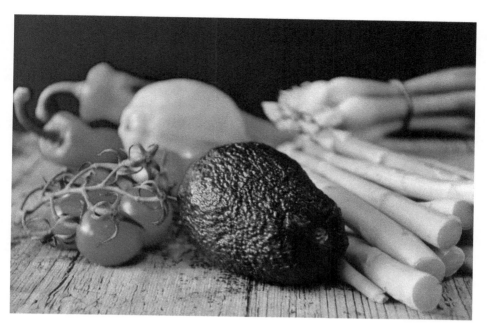

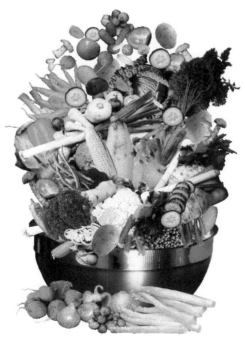

177

Lightning Source UK Ltd.
Milton Keynes UK
UKHW020743030621
384855UK00001B/256